Healthy Bones & Joints

Healthy Bones & Joints

A Natural Approach to Treating Arthritis, Osteoporosis, Tendinitis, Myalgia, and Bursitis

David Hoffmann
B. S c., F.N.I.M.H.

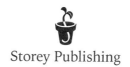

Storey Publishing

*The mission of Storey Publishing is to serve our customers by
publishing practical information that encourages
personal independence in harmony with the environment.*

This publication is intended to provide educational information for the
reader on the covered subject. It is not intended to take the place of per-
sonalized medical counseling, diagnosis, and treatment from a trained
health professional.

Edited by Deborah Balmuth and Robin Catalano
Cover design and production and text design by Betty Kodela
Text production by Susan Bernier and Jennifer Jepson Smith
Illustration on page 2 by Alison Kolesar; all other illustrations by Beverly
 Duncan, Brigita Fuhrmann, Sarah Brill, Mallory Lake, Bobbi Angell,
 Louise Riotte, Charles Joslin, and Regina Hughes
Indexed by Jon Lewis, Editype

The information in this book is true and complete to the best of our knowledge.
All recommendations are made without guarantee on the part of the author or
Storey Publishing. The author and publisher disclaim any liability in connection
with the use of this information. For additional information please contact Storey
Publishing, 210 MASS MoCA Way, North Adams, MA 01247.
 Storey books are available for special premium and promotional uses and for cus-
tomized editions. For further information, please call 1-800-793-9396.

Printed in the United States by Versa Press
10 9 8 7 6 5

Library of Congress Cataloging-in-Publication Data

Hoffmann, David, 1951–
    Healthy bones and joints: a natural approach to treating arthritis, osteoporosis,
    tendinitis, myalgia, and bursitis / David Hoffmann.
        p. cm. — (A Storey medicinal herb guide)
    Includes index.
    ISBN 978-1-58017-253-0
    1. Herbs — Therapeutic use. 2. Bones — Diseases — Alternative treatment.
    3. Joints — Diseases — Alternative treatment.   I. Title.   II. Medicinal herb guide
RM666.H33 H624 2000
616.7'06 — dc21   00-038791

CONTENTS

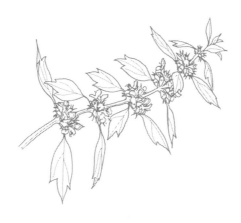

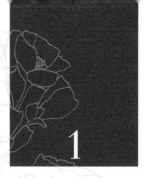

THE BODY'S FOUNDATION

The skeleton, connective tissue, muscles, and joints hold us together, enable us to stand and move, and give us our form. The musculoskeletal system is used — and misused — a lot, and it is the victim of much wear and tear. While genetically based weaknesses can play a role in musculoskeletal problems, the health of these bones and tissues depends not only on their use but also on the body's inner environment, its metabolism, diet, and lifestyle.

To a certain extent, the body's structural system can be adjusted and problems can be corrected. For example, when pain or other problems are due to skeletal misalignments, much can be done with the help of osteopathy or chiropractic. It's not uncommon for misalignments to be so extreme that they affect neurologic functions, the organs, or the harmony of the body as a whole. Alternative treatments, such as rolfing, the Alexander technique, and Feldenkrais, may be beneficial, but these therapies will not fix any underlying problems.

In many cases, the health of the bones and joints depends on the health of the body as a whole. Only as long as the inner environment and metabolism are in harmony can the body's structural system work as efficiently as it should. If, for example, the body's biochemical and metabolic processes are out of tune, the body will be under a great deal of strain as it attempts to remove wastes and toxins. If this condition lasts for some years (which it often does, and it generally goes unnoticed), toxins can build up in the connective tissue of the joints, sowing the seeds for the development of rheumatism and arthritis. This is especially true of people who have a genetic predisposition to these conditions. But herbal medicine has much to offer in the treatment of these and other chronic and degenerative ailments.

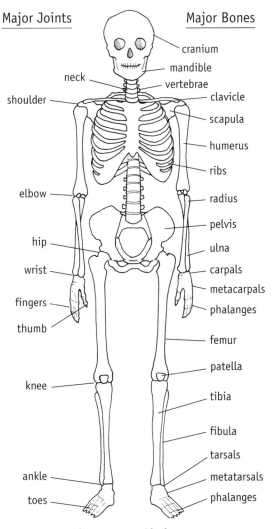

Major Joints — Major Bones

cranium
mandible
neck
vertebrae
shoulder
clavicle
scapula
humerus
ribs
elbow
radius
hip
pelvis
wrist
ulna
fingers
carpals
metacarpals
phalanges
thumb
femur
patella
knee
tibia
fibula
tarsals
ankle
metatarsals
toes
phalanges

The Human Skeleton

WHAT ARE RHEUMATIC DISEASES?

More than 100 conditions are classified as rheumatic diseases. They have in common symptoms such as pain, stiffness, and swelling in the joints and the supporting structures, such as the muscles, tendons, ligaments, and bones. Some of these diseases can also affect other parts of the body.

The term *arthritis* is often used to describe all rheumatic diseases, but this is incorrect. *Arthritis* actually means joint inflammation — that is, swelling, redness, heat, and pain, which may be caused by tissue injury or diseases of the joints. But the many kinds of arthritis comprise only a small portion of rheumatic diseases. Some rheumatic diseases instead affect the body's connective tissues. Others, known as autoimmune diseases, occur when some type of imbalance in the immune system causes it to harm the body's own healthy tissues.

In subsequent chapters, we will look at several rheumatic diseases and their treatments in some detail. But here is a quick list of the most common rheumatic diseases:

Ankylosing spondylitis. This condition, which primarily affects the spine, causes excess friction on certain joints and can lead to osteoarthritis in the hips, shoulders, and knees. The tendons and ligaments around the bones and joints in the spine become inflamed, resulting in pain and stiffness, especially in the lower back. Ankylosing spondylitis tends to affect people in late adolescence or early adulthood.

Bursitis. When the bursae, the fluid-filled sacs that cushion a joint and reduce friction during movement, become inflamed, we refer to the condition as bursitis. It may be caused by arthritis, injuries, or infections. Bursitis is painful and may limit the movement of nearby joints.

Fibromyalgia. This condition causes pain and stiffness in the muscles and other tissues that support and move bones and joints. People with fibromyalgia have pain and localized tender points in the muscles and tendons, particularly those of the neck, spine, shoulders, and hips.

Gout. This type of arthritis results from deposits of needle-like crystals of uric acid in the connective tissues, joint spaces, or both. Uric acid is a normal breakdown product of purines, which are present in body tissues and many foods. Usually, uric acid passes through the kidneys and is eliminated in the urine. When the concentration of uric acid in the blood rises above normal levels, crystals may begin to form in the tendons, ligaments, and cartilage of the joints. These crystals irritate the tissues, causing inflammation, swelling, and pain. The joints most commonly affected are those in the big toe.

Osteoarthritis. Also known as degenerative joint disease, osteoarthritis is the most common form of arthritis. It affects more than 20 million adults in the United States. It primarily affects cartilage, the tissue that cushions the ends of bones within a joint. Osteoarthritis occurs when cartilage begins to fray, wear, and decay. In extreme cases, the cartilage may wear away entirely, allowing the joint's bones to rub against each other. Friction can also cause spurs, or pointy bulges of bone, to form at the edges of the joint. Osteoarthritis often causes pain, stiffness, reduced range of motion, and an overall loss of function.

Psoriatic arthritis. This form of arthritis occurs in some people with psoriasis, a common skin disorder that results in scaling and flaking skin. Psoriatic arthritis often affects the joints at the ends of the fingers. It may be accompanied by changes in the fingernails and toenails. Some people also experience spinal problems.

Rheumatoid arthritis. This is an inflammatory disease of the lining of a joint. It results in pain, stiffness, swelling, deformity, and loss of function. The inflammation generally affects the joints in the hands and feet and tends to occur equally on both sides of the body. This symmetry helps distinguish rheumatoid arthritis from other forms of arthritis. About 2.1 million Americans have rheumatoid arthritis.

Systemic lupus erythematosus. Also known as lupus or SLE, this is an autoimmune disease — that is, it occurs when the immune system mistakenly attacks the body's tissues. It results in inflammation and may damage the joints, skin, kidneys, heart, lungs, blood vessels, and brain.

Tendinitis. This condition is an inflammation of the tendons, which are tough cords of tissue that connect muscles to bones. It's usually caused by overuse, injury, or other rheumatic conditions. Tendinitis is painful and often restricts the movement of nearby joints.

ARTHRITIS AND PAIN

Pain is the body's warning system. The International Association for the Study of Pain defines pain as an unpleasant experience associated with actual or potential tissue damage. Neurons, which are specialized cells that transmit pain signals, are located throughout the skin and other body tissues. They respond to injury or tissue damage by sending out chemical signals of pain. For example, when a knife comes in contact with the skin, the neurons in the skin send out chemical signals that travel through nerves in the spinal cord to the brain, where they are interpreted as pain.

The pain of arthritis can be acute or chronic. Acute pain is temporary; it can last only a few seconds or longer but gradually wanes as healing occurs. This type of pain can be caused by burns, cuts, and bone fractures. Chronic pain, on the other hand, ranges from mild to severe and can last a lifetime.

Arthritic pain has many causes. For example, it may occur when the synovial membrane that lines joints, tendons, and ligaments is inflamed. Muscle strain and fatigue are other culprits. But usually, the pain is caused by a combination of factors.

Pain varies greatly from person to person, but the reasons why aren't clearly understood. Factors that contribute to arthritic pain include swelling in the joint, the amount of heat present, and damage that has occurred in the joint. In addition, physical activity affects pain differently from person to person. Some people have the most pain when they first get out of bed in the morning, while others develop pain only after prolonged use of the joint. Each individual has a different tolerance for pain, due to both physical and emotional factors.

Treating with Over-the-Counter Medication

Several over-the-counter pain relievers can be helpful for addressing the discomfort of acute bone and joint pain. The drugs you use depend on the specific symptoms and the nature of the illness; there is no one-size-fits-all cure for these conditions.

For example, osteoarthritis typically involves little inflammation, so it can often be relieved with acetaminophen (such as Tylenol). This drug relieves pain but has little effect on swelling. Rheumatoid arthritis, on the contrary, does involve painful inflammation. For this reason, aspirin, ibuprofen (such as Motrin or Advil), or other nonsteroidal anti-inflammatory drugs (NSAIDs) are a better choice.

NSAIDs Can Cause Damage

NSAIDs are the most commonly used medications in the United States. They are used to treat pain, fever, and many types of inflammation. Unfortunately, NSAIDs are not without side effects, some of which can be quite serious. Every year, for example, almost 9,000 Americans die from gastrointestinal bleeding, a common side effect of NSAIDs. The full range of side effects includes:

- **Gastrointestinal effects,** such as heartburn, dyspepsia, diarrhea, constipation, abdominal pain, nausea, stomatitis, decreased appetite, and vomiting
- **Central nervous system symptoms,** including headache, insomnia, dizziness, drowsiness, tinnitus (ringing in the

REDUCING THE SIDE EFFECTS OF NSAIDS

Several simple steps can be taken when you're using NSAIDs:

• Take them with food and several glasses of water to help reduce gastrointestinal discomfort.

• Don't lie down within 30 minutes of the dose; this minimizes irritation of the delicate tissue of and near the cardiac sphincter.

• Do not take NSAIDs for chronic arthritis pain if you are elderly; have a history of peptic ulcer disease or cardiovascular disease; smoke tobacco; drink alcohol heavily; use NSAIDs heavily; or take other medications, such as warfarin (an anticoagulant) or prednisone (a steroid). These are all risk factors for gastric ulceration. Consult your physician before using NSAIDs to control arthritis pain.

ears), confusion, and weakness
• **Visual problems,** most commonly loss of visual acuity or blurred or double vision
• **Skin discomfort** from itching, rashes, photosensitivity reactions, eruptions, and hives
• **Cardiovascular effects,** such as edema, palpitations, and fast heartbeat
• **Genitourinary troubles,** including burning or painful urination, vaginal bleeding, blood in urine, and cystitis

NSAIDs can also cause much more serious problems, including ulcers, heart irregularities, kidney problems (especially in the elderly), serious skin disorders, anemia, and liver conditions, such as jaundice.

Using Prescription Drugs

A number of prescription drugs can help cases of rheumatic diseases that have not responded to over-the-counter drugs. For rheumatoid arthritis, for instance, commonly used prescription drugs include methotrexate, hydroxychloroquine, penicillamine, and gold injections. These drugs are thought to influence and correct the abnormalities of the immune system that are responsible for causing the problems. These agents may have serious side effects, and their use always requires monitoring by a physician.

Powerful anti-inflammatory drugs called corticosteroids, such as prednisone, may be used for many rheumatic conditions because they decrease inflammation and suppress the immune system. The corticosteroids are often very effective, but their frequent side effects limit their use. The short-term side effects, such as swelling, increased appetite, weight gain, and emotional swings, usually resolve when people stop taking the drugs. Long-term side effects, which may not be reversible, include stretch marks, excessive hair growth, osteoporosis, high blood pressure, damage to the arteries, high blood sugar levels, infections, and cataracts.

THE BUILDING BLOCKS OF A TREATMENT PROGRAM

The long-term goal in the treatment of rheumatic diseases is to help the person cope with the chronic, often disabling disease. The condition can create a cycle of pain, depression, and stress that is difficult to break out of. But if the patient becomes an active participant in his or her health care, the cycle is easier to break.

Several simple methods are available that will stop pain for short periods of time. Although the relief is temporary, it can improve mobility, even helping an arthritis sufferer complete tasks such as exercise.

Diet

A well-balanced diet is an important part of any treatment plan. Along with providing essential nutrients, a healthy diet — in conjunction with exercise — will help you manage your body

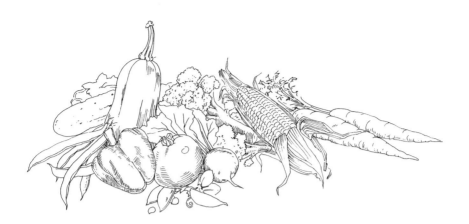

weight. This is important because extra weight puts unnecessary pressure on some joints and can aggravate arthritis.

Diet is especially important for people who have gout. If you suffer from this disease, avoid alcohol and foods that are high in purines, such as organ meats, sardines, anchovies, and meat-based gravies. The body converts purine to uric acid, an excess of which can lead to gout.

One cause of rheumatism and arthritis may be an accumulation of toxins or waste products in the affected tissues. This accumulation may occur when people eat foods that are wrong for their bodies (because of food sensitivities and allergies) or foods that have been so processed and adulterated that they simply aren't healthful.

Here are general guidelines for foods to avoid if you have a rheumatic disease:

- Foods that cause the body to have any unpleasant reaction. This includes foods that cause digestive discomfort, such as cramping or excessive gas. The best foods are those that are fresh and free of additives and preservatives.
- Gluten, a component of wheat, is a leading culprit in food allergies.
- Dairy products.
- Red meat and eggs.
- Overly acidic foods, such as vinegar and pickles.

- Foods that are rich in oxalic acid, such as rhubarb, gooseberries, and black and red currants.
- Coffee, black tea, alcohol, or anything that includes black grapes, refined sugar, and salt.

Conversely, these foods may be beneficial for a rheumatic condition:

- Fruits, including citrus. Despite their high acid content, citrus fruits seem to have an alkaline action on the metabolism. And they're an essential part of a healthy diet.
- Vegetables, particularly green and root vegetables, should be eaten in abundance. According to scientists, these foods contain compounds that can minimize the tissue damage associated with stress and aging.
- Water; drink about 2 quarts a day. Fluids help flush toxins from the body. Drink water that has a low mineral content and, if you need to, mix in a little apple juice or apple cider vinegar to make it more palatable.

In addition to these beneficial foods, take 500 mg of supplemental vitamin C per day. This vitamin helps protect tissues throughout the body, including those in the joints. While you should avoid red meat and eggs, fish and white meat are acceptable.

Glucosamine Sulfate

Glucosamine sulfate can help ease joint problems through a mechanism known as chondroprotection. Chondroprotection is a means of enhancing the reconstruction and self-healing of joint cartilage.

Glucosamine is an amino sugar, a molecule composed of an amino acid and a simple sugar. The body uses about 20 different amino sugars, either as sources of energy or as ingredients for the assembly of tissue components. Amino sugars are the structural basis of connective tissue and lubricating fluids.

GLUCOSAMINE AND CHONDROITIN COMBINATIONS

Commercial glucosamine sulfate supplements are often combined with chondroitin sulfate. Chondroitin is also a glycosaminoglycan (GAG) and is a major constituent of cartilage. This GAG provides structure, holds water and nutrients, and allows other molecules to move through the cartilage; this action is important, since there is no blood supply to cartilage. But there is no strong evidence to support the use of glucosamine and chondroitin in combination, especially since scientists still question whether chondroitin is absorbed when taken orally. If you decide to try this combination supplement, the typical dosage for osteoarthritis is 400 mg. three times a day.

Just as amino acids are the building blocks of proteins, amino sugars are the building blocks of very large molecules called glycosaminoglycans (GAGs), or mucopolysaccharides. GAGs are spongy, water-holding molecules that form the gel-like matrix found in all connective tissue and mucous membranes. Essentially, they are the "glue" that holds us together. Glucosamine macromolecules are the basic substrate of cartilage, ligaments, tendons, and bones.

Connective tissue is constantly being broken down and then replaced or restructured, creating a continuous demand for glucosamine. The average diet is not a good source of glucosamine, so this substance is synthesized by the body from glucose and the amino acid glutamine. The body normally can produce enough glucosamine, but under some conditions — severe physical and emotional stress, for example, as well as simple aging — production may be impaired. In many rheumatic diseases, a lack of glycoproteins or other substances based on amino sugars has been found. Osteoarthritis is an example of these diseases.

Some evidence suggests that taking glucosamine sulfate supplements may stimulate synthesis of the missing glycoproteins. In one study, the effects of taking glucosamine sulfate were compared with those of taking ibuprofen and indomethacin (a prescription anti-inflammatory drug). In people with osteoarthritis, the drugs relieved the symptoms faster than glucosamine sulfate did, but they also had a negative long-term effect on cartilage and the course of the disease. People taking glucosamine sulfate experienced relief after only 2 weeks of treatment. Those who took it for 8 weeks had long-term relief, even after they stopped taking it.

If you decide to try glucosamine sulfate supplements for your joint condition, don't expect instant results; it takes 2 to 8 weeks to fully stimulate the body's synthesis of the missing macromolecules. The suggested dosage for the treatment of osteoarthritis is 500 mg three times per day.

Heat and Cold

Applications of both heat and cold have been shown to help reduce the pain and inflammation of arthritis. Studies have shown that heat and cold therapies are equally effective in reducing pain. However, deciding when to use heat or cold depends on the condition being treated.

Heat increases blood flow and improves flexibility and pain tolerance in sore joints. Heat can be applied in many ways. Physical therapists often apply melted paraffin wax to the skin over the affected area, and they also employ microwave and ultrasound heat treatments. But you can apply some heat treatments at home.

Moist heat, such as a warm bath or shower, and dry heat in the form of a heating pad can be effective. Apply any of these treatments to the painful area of the joint for about 15 minutes. Heating for longer periods does not improve the condition. In addition, heat is not recommended for people with acutely inflamed joints. This includes patients with gout; heat increases circulation, thus aggravating inflammation. However, heat is often used around the shoulder to relax tight tendons before stretching exercises.

Cold applications numb the nerves around the joint, reducing pain. This therapy also relieves inflammation and muscle spasms. Cold therapy can involve cold packs, ice massage, cold-water soaking, or over-the-counter sprays and ointments that cool the skin and joints.

For an easy home treatment, wrap an ice pack (or a bag of frozen vegetables) in a towel and place it on the sore area for about 15 minutes. This is recommended for acutely inflamed joints; it will help reduce both swelling and pain. People who have Raynaud's phenomenon, a circulatory illness, should not use this technique because it causes local vasoconstriction that dramatically aggravates the condition.

Weight Reduction

Weight loss is one of the most effective ways to both relieve and help prevent joint pain. Excess weight puts stress on the knees, hips, back, and other joints. In one study, overweight women who lost an average of 11 pounds substantially reduced the development of osteoarthritis in their knees. Even when osteoarthritis has already affected one joint, weight reduction will reduce the chance that it will occur in another.

ASSISTIVE DEVICES

Splints and braces are common assistive devices for treating arthritis pain. Both devices support weakened joints, allowing them to rest. Some assistive devices prevent the joint from moving, while others allow for some movement. Still other devices ease the pain by cushioning and taking pressure off a joint. For example, using a cane will reduce some of the weight placed on an arthritic leg joint. A shoe insert helps ease the foot or knee pain associated with walking by correcting improper angles, such as supinating arches.

Use a splint or brace only after your health-care practitioner has fit you for one and shown you how to put it on — and explained how long you should wear it. Incorrect use can cause stiffness, pain, and even joint damage.

Hydrotherapy, Mobilization Therapy, and Relaxation Therapy

Many physical and mental therapies can help people deal with joint pain and can help slow the progression of the illness. Three of the most popular techniques are hydrotherapy, mobilization therapy, and relaxation therapy.

Hydrotherapy involves exercising or relaxing in warm water. It helps relax tense muscles and relieve pain. Exercising in a large pool (one with enough room for full movement) is easier than exercising on land because water provides buoyancy that takes some of the weight off painful joints. This type of exercise improves muscle strength and joint movement.

Mobilization therapies include traction (gentle, steady pulling), massage, and manipulation (using the hands to restore normal movement to stiff joints). When used by a trained professional, these methods can help control pain, increase joint motion, and improve muscle and tendon flexibility. Although massage increases blood flow and warmth to stressed areas, it may cause pain around the affected joints. Work only with a massage therapist who has experience treating the condition.

Relaxation therapy is used to help people relax muscle tension; this, in turn, reduces pain around the affected joints. In progressive relaxation, people are taught to tighten one muscle group, slowly release the tension, and then repeat the process with another group. You can learn about relaxation therapy from your doctor or physical therapist.

Exercise

For most people with bone or joint problems, gentle exercise is among the best possible therapies. Exercise reduces joint pain and stiffness and increases flexibility, muscle strength, and endurance. It also helps people lose weight and contributes to an

How to Start an Exercise Program

Before embarking on a new exercise program, be sure to consult your doctor and physical therapist. In addition, follow these general guidelines:

- Always begin with stretching exercises.
- Warm up with range-of-motion exercises.
- When doing strengthening exercises, start slowly with small weights.
- Progress slowly; do not increase the number of repetitions or length of time you exercise until you have worked through the previous level for several weeks without pain. Check with your physical therapist if you're unsure.
- Use cold packs after exercising.
- When you're able, add aerobic exercise to your program.
- Ease back if your joints become painful, inflamed, or red.
- Choose the exercise program you enjoy the most; you are more likely to stick with the plan if you like what you're doing.

improved sense of well-being. Of course, exercise is only one part of a comprehensive arthritis treatment plan — a plan that may also include rest and relaxation, dietary modifications, proper joint movement, and pain relief medications.

The amount and type of exercise needed varies widely, depending on which joints are involved, the amount of inflammation, the stability of the joints, and whether there has been a joint replacement. When you are using exercise to relieve arthritis or other bone or joint problems, it's important to work with a physician who is skilled in rehabilitative medicine. It's also helpful to work with a physical therapist who is familiar with the needs of the arthritic patient.

Three types of exercise are best for people with arthritis:

- **Range-of-motion exercises,** such as stretching, help maintain normal joint movement, relieve stiffness, and improve flexibility.
- **Strengthening exercises,** such as light weightlifting, maintain or increase muscle strength. Strong muscles support and protect arthritic joints.
- **Aerobic or endurance exercises,** such as walking and swimming, improve cardiovascular fitness and help control weight.

Your physical therapist or physician will design an appropriate home exercise program and teach you about joint protection, physical energy conservation, and proper body mechanics — for example, how best to use your body when picking up a heavy box.

2

USING HERBS AS MEDICINE

The different varieties of arthritis are perhaps the most significant inflammatory conditions to affect humanity. *Arthritis,* which simply means "joint inflammation," is a general term for approximately 100 recognized diseases that produce either inflammation of connective tissues, particularly in joints, or non-inflammatory degeneration of these tissues. But because these diseases often affect other body structures, the terms *connective tissue disease* and *rheumatism* are also used. Causes of these disorders include immune-system reactions, the wear and tear of aging, and chronic injury, but research suggests that the nervous system may be equally involved.

Throughout the world, herbal medicine is used to treat arthritis. Used within a broad holistic context (see chapter 1 for more information), herbal medicine works with the body to promote improvement of the condition while alleviating pain and discomfort. But simply taking anti-inflammatory and anti-rheumatic remedies is not enough; arthritis therapy must also focus on liver function, circulation, and toxin elimination as well as lifestyle changes.

TAKING A HOLISTIC APPROACH

We need not look into the differences between the various kinds of arthritis in too much depth. It is arguable whether a differential diagnosis is even necessary for holistic treatment. But what is necessary to recognize is the general and individual causes and the influences of a person's genetic framework. The aim of holistic treatment is to bring the person's body and mind into a state of balance so that the body can take care of the symptoms.

The Role of Friction

An important consideration in the treatment of arthritic conditions is friction. *Webster's Tenth Collegiate Dictionary* defines friction as "resistance to relative motion between two bodies in contact; disagreement." The changes in the joints that are caused by arthritis ultimately make the bones rub together, which, of course, causes pain. But in arthritis, there is often a long history of friction leading up to the physical change in the joints.

For instance, a farmer may develop osteoarthritis in the shoulder on which he has carried hay bales every morning for many years. Sometimes the joint friction is the result of friction in life, as when the muscles of a person who has endured constant stress bind the joints together too tightly. When looking at the roots of rheumatic and arthritic problems, it's easy to see the large role played by friction.

When trying to create the right internal environment for healing, as much attention must be paid to emotional and mental harmony as to diet and herbal medicine. If you have an outlook that is tight, defensive, and lacking in vulnerability and openness, the rheumatism will feed off your tension. But if you allow yourself to relax, interact with others, and express your emotions and beliefs, you will go a long way toward self-healing.

How Herbs Can Help

Through the use of appropriate herbs and other techniques that support and aid the whole body, it is possible to cleanse the entire inner environment and remove the source of the rheumatic or arthritic development. Such a treatment takes time, since degenerative processes cannot be reversed in a couple of weeks. But when the right combination treatment is used, it's not uncommon for arthritis patients to make statements like "I feel better already" even before the actual symptoms of pain or stiffness are gone.

With rheumatic and arthritic conditions, more so than with any other condition, it is essential to treat the whole person. Otherwise, improvement will be only slight or temporary. When the unique individual picture is taken into account, healing is promoted. For example, does your digestive system need help in any way? Are your kidneys working well? Is there too much stress in your life? How good is your diet? Answers to these and other questions will help you and your health care practitioner design an herbal program that meets your unique needs.

A great deal of pharmaceutical research has gone into analyzing the active constituents of herbs to find out how and why they work. However, a much older and far more relevant approach is to categorize herbs by the kinds of problems they can treat. In some cases the action is due to a specific chemical in the herb, while in other cases it might be due to a complex synergistic interaction between a number of the plant's constituents. It's always best to view the herb as a whole; an understanding of the chemistry is simply an aid in prescription.

Because of herb chemistry's wonderful complexity, a single herb might produce a range of responses in the human body. For example, chamomile contains several active components in its volatile oil, in addition to nonvolatile flavonoids (aromatic compounds that often act as antioxidants and anti-inflammatories) and sesquiterpenes (hydrocarbon compounds). This cornucopia of chemistry allows chamomile to act as an anti-inflammatory, antispasmodic, antimicrobial, and relaxing nervine all in one!

Herbal Actions Defined

Some herb constituents produce certain actions that are uniquely suited for treating digestive system problems. We group these actions into the following categories:

Adaptogen. Increases resistance and resilience to stress, enabling the body to adjust to the problem. Adaptogens seem to work by supporting the adrenal glands.

Alterative. Gradually restores proper functioning of the body, increasing health and vitality. Some alteratives support natural waste elimination through the kidneys, liver, lungs, or skin. Others stimulate digestive function or are antimicrobial, and others just work!

Anticatarrhal. Helps the body remove excess mucus in the sinuses or other parts of the body. Mucus itself is not a problem, but the body may produce too much in response to an infection or as a way to get rid of excess carbohydrates.

Anti-inflammatory. Soothes or reduces inflammation. Anti-inflammatories work in many different ways, but they rarely inhibit the natural inflammatory reaction directly. Rather, they support the body as it is working.

Antimicrobial. Helps the body destroy or resist pathogenic microorganisms. Some antimicrobial herbs have antiseptic properties, but these herbs generally work by strengthening the body's natural immunity.

Antispasmodic. Eases muscle cramps and helps relieve muscular tension. Many antispasmodic agents are also nervines, and these agents relieve psychological tension in addition to physical tension.

Astringent. Has a bracing action on mucous membranes, skin, and other tissue. Because of chemicals called tannins, astringents bind with protein molecules, thus reducing irritation and inflammation and creating barriers against infections. These herbs are helpful for healing wounds and burns.

Bitter. Has a special role in preventive medicine. The taste of a bitter herb triggers a sensory response in the central nervous system, and this causes the intestine to release digestive hormones. Bitters are used to stimulate the appetite and the flow of digestive juices. They also aid the liver in detoxification, increase bile flow, and stimulate self-repair mechanisms in the gut.

Cardiac remedy. A general term for herbal remedies that benefit the heart. Some cardiac remedies in this group are powerful cardioactive agents, such as foxglove; others are gentler, safer herbs, such as hawthorn and motherwort.

Carminative. Stimulates the digestive system, soothes the gut wall, reduces any inflammation, eases griping pains, and helps remove gas from the digestive tract.

Demulcent. Soothes and protects irritated or inflamed tissue. Demulcents reduce irritation down the whole length of the bowel, reduce sensitivity to potentially corrosive gastric acids, and help prevent diarrhea. They also reduce the muscle spasms that cause colic and the bronchial tension that causes coughing.

Diaphoretic. Promotes perspiration, helping the skin eliminate waste from the body. Some diaphoretics produce observable sweat; others aid normal perspiration. Diaphoretics often promote dilation of surface capillaries, which improves circulation. They support the work of the kidneys by increasing cleansing through the skin.

Diuretic. Increases production and elimination of urine. In herbal medicine, with its ancient traditions, the term is often applied to herbs that have a beneficial action on the urinary system as a whole. Diuretics help the body eliminate waste and support the process of inner cleansing.

Emmenagogue. Stimulates menstrual flow and activity. The term is also applied to remedies that normalize and tone the female reproductive system.

Expectorant. Stimulates the removal of mucus from the lungs and acts as a tonic for the respiratory system. Stimulating expectorants "irritate" the bronchioles, causing expulsion of material. Relaxing expectorants soothe bronchial spasms and loosen mucous secretions, relieving dry, irritating coughs.

Hepatic. Aids the liver by toning; strengthening; and, in some cases, increasing the flow of bile. Hepatics are important because the liver plays a fundamental role in the body.

Hypotensive. Lowers abnormally elevated blood pressure.

Laxative. Stimulates bowel movements. Laxatives should not be used over a long period; diet, general health, and stress levels should all be closely considered when constipation persists.

Nervine. All three types of nervines help the nervous system. Nervine tonics strengthen and restore the nervous system, nervine relaxants ease anxiety and tension by soothing both body and mind, and nervine stimulants directly stimulate nerve activity.

Rubefacient. Generates a localized increase in blood flow when applied to the skin, encouraging healing, cleansing, and nourishment. Rubefacients are often used to ease the pain and swelling of arthritic joints.

Tonic. Nurtures and invigorates. Tonics are truly gifts from nature to a suffering humanity. To ask how they work is to ask how life itself works!

Vulnerary. Promotes wound healing. Used mainly to describe herbs that heal skin lesions. They also work for internal wounds, such as stomach ulcers.

In most cases, successful herbal treatment of musculoskeletal illness is based on support for the whole body; this is because systemic factors are often the foundation for degenerative conditions. Thus, the most effective antirheumatics are primarily alteratives, diuretics, or other herbs that have beneficial effects for the body as a whole. Anti-inflammatory herbs serve to reduce symptoms but do not usually improve the disease process. An exception to this rule is a case of arthritis in which an active

COMMON HERBAL ANTIRHEUMATICS

Anti-Inflammatories	Alteratives	Diuretics	Circulatory Stimulants
Angelica	Bogbean	Bearberry	Bayberry
Birch	Burdock	Boneset	Cayenne
Bogbean	Devil's claw	Celery seed	Ginger
Celery seed	Guaiacum	Dandelion	Horseradish
Devil's claw	Kelp	Gravel root	Mustard
Feverfew	Mountain grape	Parsley	Prickly ash
Guaiacum	Nettle	Yarrow	Rosemary
Meadowsweet	Poke		
White poplar	Sarsaparilla		**Antispasmodics**
Wild yam	Yellow dock		Black cohosh
Willow bark			Cramp bark
Wintergreen			

inflammation is worsening the pathological changes in the bone tissue; in this situation, anti-inflammatories are very important.

ANTIRHEUMATICS

Many herbs are reputed to prevent, relieve, and even cure some rheumatic conditions. The following long (but far from complete) list of antirheumatics includes alteratives, anti-inflammatories, rubefacients, diuretics, stimulants, and digestives; thus, you may choose an herb depending on the needs of your body. These remedies have been shown over centuries to provide relief for people with a variety of rheumatic conditions, although not necessarily because they have a direct effect on the disease or the musculoskeletal system. While the primary action of an antirheumatic is important, it is usually the synergy of the plant's various actions that makes these herbs successful.

ALTERATIVES

The alterative herbs gradually restore the proper functioning of the body and increase health and vitality. This may sound a bit unclear, but that's because the mode of action of these herbs is not completely understood. Nonetheless, the value of these herbs in holistic health care cannot be doubted.

In broad terms, alteratives change the body's metabolic processes, helping the tissues deal with a wide range of functions, from nutrition to elimination. Many alteratives improve the body's ability to eliminate wastes through the kidneys, liver, lungs, or skin. Others work by stimulating digestive function, while some are antimicrobial. Others just work!

Alteratives are often referred to as *blood cleansers,* a term that hints at much but says little. Indeed, if the blood were in need of cleansing, we would have a major medical emergency afoot. But immunological research on plant products is leading to some interesting thoughts about the actions of alteratives. Saponins, which are plant glucosides, are known to have many properties — including strengthening the immune system. They also appear to help increase the production of white cell macrophages of the mononuclear phagocyte system (MPS). Since the MPS is responsible for removing much of the waste matter from the blood, we can say that it "cleanses" the blood. That sounds like classic alterative activity! Still, the specifics of plant chemical activity are the result of the whole plant — not just a few active ingredients — affecting the human body.

Alteratives can be used safely as supportive remedies for many conditions. They should be among the first choices for chronic inflammatory or degenerative conditions, such as arthritis, skin diseases, and some autoimmune problems. Most alteratives are helpful for treating arthritis, but those most commonly used are black cohosh, bogbean, celery seed, devil's claw, guaiacum, and sarsaparilla. These herbs have a cleansing action that generally revitalizes the body.

There are plants that are particularly suited for each system of the body. Here are some of the main alteratives and brief descriptions of their unique actions.

- **Circulatory system.** Cleavers, echinacea, and poke root help the body circulate fluids, including lymph, more efficiently.
- **Respiratory system.** Mullein, garlic, and goldenseal are beneficial for the lungs and the respiratory system as a whole.
- **Digestive system.** Bogbean, burdock, garlic, goldenseal, nettle, sarsaparilla, yellow dock, and quite a few other alteratives work on the liver, pancreas, and other organs of the digestive system. They have great importance in the whole of herbal medicine.
- **Urinary system.** Some of the plants that herbalists call diuretics could be described as urinary alteratives. These herbs include cleavers and nettles.
- **Reproductive system.** Black cohosh is a specific for the support of this system, although the general alteratives also have value.
- **Musculoskeletal system.** Black cohosh, bogbean, and burdock are just a few of the alteratives that are important, since they also work as antirheumatics.
- **Nervous system.** Pasque flower and red clover have a nervine action that's important for this system as a whole.

ANTI-INFLAMMATORIES

The world is abundant in plants that act as anti-inflammatories. This should come as no surprise, since ecological integration ensures that most of the biological needs of humans and other animals are met. While anti-inflammatories are rarely as powerful as steroidal drugs, they are also rarely as dangerous.

Inflammation, a process that is unpleasantly familiar to just about everyone, occurs in response to a range of traumas — from sunburn and wounds to infection and autoimmune disease. Whatever the cause, the result is basically the same. It is characterized by four main signs:

- **Warmth,** caused by the dilation of small blood vessels in the injured area and increased local blood flow.
- **Redness,** which is due to the same causes as warmth.
- **Swelling,** which is a product of protein-rich exudate that escapes from blood plasma, through blood vessels (which become more permeable during inflammation), and into the damaged tissues.
- **Pain,** a result of chemical substances (such as serotonin) or the tension of the tissue over the inflamed area.

The inflammation in an autoimmune condition, such as rheumatoid arthritis, is fundamentally the same as that in a simple infection or wound. The trigger of the reaction, however, is very different.

Traditional Western medicine places much emphasis on chemical anti-inflammatories that reduce symptoms but do not treat the disease itself. Anti-inflammatories are safe to use for the relief of pain and discomfort, but they are best used in combination with other remedies that address the underlying problem.

Herbs can reduce inflammation in a number of different ways, but they only rarely do this by inhibiting the body's natural reactions. Rather, they support and encourage the work that the body is doing. This cooperation is important because inflammation is a normal response to infection or other trauma. Through localized biochemical and tissue changes, the inflammatory reaction often brings about the changes necessary to restore health.

For the most part, unless inflammation is life-threatening, it's a mistake to inhibit it. For example, simply suppressing the symptoms of stomach inflammation does not alter the underlying problem. And since prolonged use of anti-inflammatories can even cause damage, such as stomach ulcers, pharmaceuticals are not the best method of managing inflammation. Instead, we

COMMON HERBAL ANTI-INFLAMMATORIES

Angelica	Devil's claw	Marsh mallow	Willow bark
Birch	Elder	Meadowsweet	Wintergreen
Black cohosh	Fennel	Mullein	Witch hazel
Black haw	Fenugreek	Peppermint	Yarrow
Bogbean	Goldenseal	Plantain	
Bupleurum	Guaiacum	Sage	
Calendula	Hawthorn	Shepherd's	
Celery seed	Horse chestnut	purse	
Chamomile	Hyssop	Slippery elm	
Chickweed	Lavender	St.-John's-wort	
Cleavers	Licorice	White poplar	
Cramp bark	Linden	Wild yam	

should look to herbal remedies, which offer us their inflamma-tion-reducing properties while also helping us to achieve a state of balance within the body.

Generally, herbal anti-inflammatories fall into several main groups, each of which works in a different way. However, remember that the action of any plant always involves more than the action of any specific constituent chemical. Keeping this holistic perspective in mind, let's take a look at these different groups.

Salicin–Containing Anti–Inflammatories

Many plants contain natural, aspirin-like chemicals called sal-icylates. It is worth noting that aspirin itself was originally isolated from plant sources. In fact, the name *aspirin* comes from the old botanical genus name of meadowsweet, *Spiraea*. The word *salicylate* derives from willow's Latin name, *Salix*.

Salicin-containing anti-inflammatories are quite effective for relieving arthritic pain without causing aspirin's main side effect, stomach upset. (Meadowsweet, which is rich in salicylates, can be

ANTI-INFLAMMATORIES
FOR DIFFERENT PARTS OF THE BODY

Many plants with anti-inflammatory capabilities are particularly suited to specific body systems because the herbs also have other actions. This duality allows you to nurture the health and vitality of specific body systems while reducing inflammation.

- **For the circulatory system,** choose hawthorn, horse chestnut, linden, or yarrow — all of which reduce inflammation in blood vessels.

- **For the digestive system,** particularly problems such as stomach ulcers, colitis, and hemorrhoids, try chamomile, goldenseal, licorice, marigold, peppermint, or wild yam. Demulcent herbs, such as marsh mallow, are helpful here because they are rich in mucilage and may reduce local inflammation.

- **For the urinary system,** use herbs that soothe tissues as they are passed through the kidneys and bladder. These remedies, some of which fight infection and thus reduce inflammatory reactions, include cornsilk and goldenrod.

- **For the reproductive system,** select system-specific herbs such as blue cohosh and lady's mantle.

- **For the muscles and bones,** salicylate-containing remedies will relieve the pain of overuse. Birch, meadowsweet, white poplar, and willow bark are all excellent examples. Also consider black cohosh, bogbean, devil's claw, feverfew, and wild yam.

- **For the nervous system,** try relaxing nervines, such as oat and valerian. St.-John's-wort, which is recognized as the only anti-inflammatory that is effective on nerve tissue, will help the recovery of damaged nerves.

- **For the skin,** there are many herbal choices. Arnica, calendula, chickweed, plantain, and St.-John's-wort are the most popular.

used to staunch mild stomach hemorrhage even though salicylates generally contribute to such hemorrhage.) Other plants rich in anti-inflammatory constituents include birch, black haw, willow bark, wintergreen, and many of the poplars.

Phytosterol–Containing Anti–Inflammatories

Some herbs contain chemicals that are metabolized in the body to natural steroidal molecules that fight inflammation. (Like aspirin, steroids were first isolated from plant materials.) These steroidal molecules are similar to those in allopathic medications but are safer to use. Herbs in this category include bupleurum, licorice, and wild yam.

Essential Oil–Containing Anti–Inflammatories

Many of the aromatic herbs, with their wonderful essential oils, have anti-inflammatory action. One of the best of these remedies is chamomile, which is rich in terpenes (a type of hydrocarbon), such as bisobolol and chamazulene. Calendula and St.-John's-wort are other well-known plants containing oils that soothe and reduce inflammation.

Resin–Containing Anti–Inflammatories

Many resin-containing plants reduce inflammation in some areas of the body, but they often cause inflammation in the stomach. This has limited their use, but they remain irreplaceable in the treatment of some arthritic conditions. These herbs include bogbean, devil's claw, and guaiacum.

Other Types of Anti–Inflammatories

As is typical with herbal remedies, many valuable anti-inflammatories have no clear-cut chemical basis for their actions.

But this again proves that there is more to health and well-being than pharmaceutical chemistry! Of the many remedies that fall into this "other" category, black cohosh is most prominent. Demulcent herbs frequently have an apparently anti-inflammatory effect, but they actually just soothe inflamed surfaces rather than reducing the cellular inflammatory response.

RUBEFACIENTS

When applied to the skin, rubefacients stimulate circulation; this, in turn, relieves congestion and inflammation. Rubefacients are particularly useful as ingredients in liniments for relieving muscular rheumatism and similar conditions.

Rubefacients are used topically to ease joint problems. Because they can irritate the skin, they should be used with care by people with sensitive skin and shouldn't be used at all on damaged skin.

Common Herbal Rubefacients

Cayenne
Ginger
Horseradish
Mustard
Peppermint essential oil
Ragwort
Rosemary
Wintergreen essential oil

DIURETICS

Herbs with a diuretic action help the kidneys process and eliminate metabolic wastes and toxins. They also help the body expel the by-products of inflammation. This is essential because these by-products may lie at the root of arthritis or rheumatism.

Because diuretics promote urination, you should drink plenty of water while taking them in order to avoid dehydration.

Common Herbal Diuretics

Bearberry
Boneset
Celery seed
Dandelion leaf
Gravel root
Parsley
Yarrow

CIRCULATORY STIMULANTS

Another way to cleanse the body of toxins is to stimulate the circulation. Doing this increases blood flow to muscles and joints and removes pain-causing by-products from these areas. One danger of this practice is that it may place an undue burden on the heart. Fortunately, many herbs circumvent this risk by stimulating the peripheral circulation.

Common Herbal Circulatory Stimulants

Cayenne
Ginger
Poke root
Prickly ash
Rosemary

PAIN RELIEVERS

While the herbal purist will always be reluctant to "merely" treat symptoms, the healer's art aims at relieving suffering. It may be necessary to use herbs that will reduce the often-severe pain of conditions such as rheumatism. Of course, these herbs will be used only as part of an overall treatment plan directed toward clearing the underlying problem.

Common Herbal Pain Relievers

Guaiacum
Jamaican dogwood
St.-John's-wort
Valerian

DIGESTIVE TONICS

For nutrients supporting the musculoskeletal system to be properly absorbed, the body's digestive process must work properly. The use of bitter tonics aids the entire digestive system by stimulating and supporting the digestive process.

Several tonics, including gentian, goldenseal, wormwood, and yarrow, can be used for rheumatic conditions. Should constipation be present, it may be helpful to use laxatives, especially those that support the liver. Some laxative herbs are dandelion root, rhubarb root, and yellow dock.

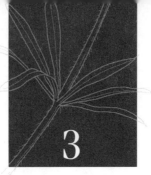

TREATING COMMON BONE AND JOINT DISEASES

Although there is a wide array of bone and joint conditions, some are so prevalent that millions of people seek treatment for them every year. Whether acute or chronic, diseases of the musculoskeletal system are almost always painful and are often debilitating. Learning to treat your particular condition with herbs — in a broader holistic context, of course — can help you reduce the intensity and frequency of your symptoms. In some cases, it may even alleviate the problem altogether.

Arthritis, which may be the most troubling of all inflammatory conditions, affects millions of people. Depending on its type, it produces inflammation of connective tissues, particularly in the joints, or noninflammatory degeneration of the tissues. Arthritis may be a result of simple physical friction, or it may be caused by an immune reaction — either because the body is fighting germs and overreacts or because the body mistakes its own tissues for invaders. In the latter case, antiself antibodies react with connective tissue and the synovial membranes, causing inflammation.

A common form of arthritis caused by autoimmune problems is rheumatoid arthritis. In most cases of rheumatoid arthritis, the synovial membranes (the inner linings of the joint capsules) are chronically inflamed. Over time, the inflammation destroys cartilage, bone, and adjacent structures.

Regardless of the underlying cause, most of these musculoskeletal conditions are best understood in the context of physical friction. As tissues in the joints are damaged, the roughened areas of bone may begin rubbing together, causing pain as well as additional damage. But herbal remedies can help, both by addressing specific symptoms of musculoskeletal disease and by treating other areas of the body that need support.

Basic Tea for Arthritis/Rheumatism

This tea is a basic mixture for rheumatic and arthritic conditions. It can be used to treat most types of musculoskeletal discomfort.

2 parts bogbean
1 part black cohosh
1 part celery seed
1 part meadowsweet

To make: Combine all ingredients. Make a decoction following the instructions on pages 103–104.
To use: Drink 1 cup (240 ml) 3 times per day for a long period; 4 to 6 weeks is a good guide.

BURSITIS AND TENDINITIS

Adjacent to joints are bursae, small sacs of connective tissue. Lined by a smooth inner surface, the bursae facilitate the gliding movements of muscles and tendons over bony prominences. Bursitis occurs when one or more bursae become inflamed, often because of pressure or a hard knock. Any bursa can be affected, but the most common types of bursitis occur in the shoulder, elbow, hip, and knee.

Bursitis is associated with strenuous activity, particularly among manual laborers and athletes. Normally sedentary people who push themselves beyond their physical limitations are also at risk for developing bursitis. Housemaid's knee is a common type of bursitis; tennis elbow is another frequently seen condition. When bursitis is chronic, it may be part of the gradual development of rheumatic problems. Read the section on rheumatism (page 40) for treatment.

Bursitis that is mild and short-term can usually be treated by applying a warm compress to the area or by applying a stimulating liniment (see Myalgia and Arthritis for more information). Both will help reduce inflammation and ease pain. If the problem continues, however, internal treatments similar to those used for myalgia and arthritis may be necessary.

Don't ignore chronic bursitis. While you may be tempted to "tough out" the pain, untreated bursitis can lead to the formation of calcium deposits in soft tissues. This may cause a permanent reduction in the range of motion of the joint.

Tendinitis is characterized by inflammation in or around a tendon, which is the fibrous tissue that connects a muscle to a bone. Tendons can withstand a lot of bending, stretching, and twisting, but overuse, disease, and traumatic injuries can cause them to become painful and inflamed. The pain can be significant and will worsen if the joint continues to be used.

Tendinitis can develop as the result of any activity, but by far the most common cause is repetitive stress — using the same joints for the same movement again and again. This type of movement happens not only in sports, but also in many types of office and manual work. Most cases of tendinitis heal in about 2 weeks, but chronic tendinitis can last more than 6 weeks, often because people remain active and don't give the tendon time to recover.

Treating with Herbs

Several types of herbs have proven helpful in the treatment of both bursitis and tendinitis:

- **Antirheumatics** usually help, but you should consider their other properties before choosing.
- **Anti-inflammatories,** such as willow bark, are helpful for symptomatic relief.
- **Antispasmodics,** such as cramp bark, reduce the muscle tension that accompanies tendinitis and bursitis.
- **Circulatory stimulants and rubefacients** help speed healing by increasing blood flow to the area.

For a topical treatment, try mixing equal parts lobelia tincture and cramp bark tincture; rub into the affected areas as needed.

Willow Bark–Cramp Bark Tincture

This combination of antirheumatics has other healing actions to offer, including anti-inflammatory (willow bark, celery seed), antispasmodic (cramp bark, celery seed), and vasodilatory (prickly ash).

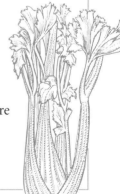

2 parts willow bark
2 parts cramp bark
2 parts celery seed
1 part prickly ash

To make: Combine all ingredients. Make a tincture following the instructions on page 104.
To use: Take 1 teaspoon (5 ml) of the tincture 3 times per day.

Lifestyle Treatments

A variety of nonherb treatments can be used to relieve tendinitis and bursitis. These treatments are primarily geared toward symptom relief, although they can also speed healing.

- Deep-heat therapy (diathermy) can alleviate the discomfort and inflammation of bursitis while soothing tense muscles, nerves, and tendons. Your physical therapist can provide the appropriate deep-heat treatment for you.
- Warming up before strenuous exercise and cooling down afterward is the most effective way to avoid tendinitis and other strains affecting the bones, muscles, and ligaments.
- Adequate rest is crucial. Returning too soon to the activity that caused the injury can lead to chronic tendinitis, torn tendons, or continuing bursitis.

The goals of any bursitis or tendinitis treatment are to restore painless movement to the joint and maintain strength in surrounding muscles while giving the damaged tissue time to heal.

THE RICE PROGRAM

This regimen is the mainstay in the treatment of tendinitis and other soft-tissue injuries. RICE stands for Rest, Ice, Compression, and Elevation.

- **Rest** is mainly a matter of remembering not to use the joint, especially for the same action that injured it.
- **Ice** can be applied in the form of a bag of frozen vegetables if no ice pack is handy.
- **Compression** is best provided by a sports bandage. Wrap the area snugly, but not so that the bandage is painfully tight.
- **Elevation** means reducing local blood pressure by raising the injured area. For example, put your ankle on a footstool or lift your elbow onto a table when you're sitting or lying down.

GOUT

Gout, one of the most painful rheumatic diseases, occurs when deposits of needle-like crystals of uric acid form in the connective tissue, joint spaces, or both. An attack of acute gouty arthritis occurs when the crystals are ingested by white blood cells. The cells release enzymes that cause inflammation.

Gout accounts for about 5 percent of all cases of arthritis. A condition called pseudogout (also known as calcium pyrophosphate deposition disease or chondrocalcinosis), which is also triggered by crystal deposits, produces symptoms very similar to those of gout. However, the crystals in pseudogout are formed from calcium pyrophosphate dihydrate rather than uric acid.

Uric acid is a naturally occurring substance formed from the chemical breakdown of purines. Purines' bases are found in DNA, our genetic material. When cells die and release DNA from their chromosomes, purines are released and then converted into uric acid. Uric acid is excreted in the urine and, to a lesser extent, from the intestinal tract. But if the body increases its production of uric acid, or if the kidneys do not eliminate enough uric acid from the body, levels of uric acid begin to rise. This condition is called hyperuricemia.

In some cases, hyperuricemia occurs when people eat too many high-purine foods, such as liver, dried beans and peas, anchovies, and meat-based gravies. High purine levels alone aren't dangerous, but if the extra uric acid should precipitate into crystals, gout may result. Only 1 in 20 cases of hyperuricemia develops into gout.

The main symptom of gout is extreme joint pain, often in the big toe; this condition is called podagra. Occasionally, large deposits of uric acid called tophi appear as lumps under the skin around the joints or the rim of the ear. Uric acid crystals can also collect in the kidneys, causing kidney stones.

A handful of factors can put you at risk for hyperuricemia and gout. These include:

- **Genetics.** Between 6 and 18 percent of people with gout have a family history of the disease.
- **Being overweight.** Excessive food intake increases the body's production of uric acid.
- **Alcohol consumption.** Heavy drinking may interfere with the removal of uric acid from the body.
- **Purine-rich diet.** This type of diet can both cause and aggravate gout.
- **An enzyme defect.** Some people cannot properly break down purines because of an enzyme defect that interferes with the process.
- **Exposure to lead.** This substance inhibits the secretion of uric acid.

Treating with Herbs

Diuretics can play a pivotal role in controlling gout because they help flush uric acid from the body. Anti-inflammatories may also help, but generally they're not very effective. They are not recommended because the body's inflammatory response is a natural reaction to the crystals.

MEDICINES ALSO INCREASE YOUR RISK

For a variety of reasons, several prescription and over-the-counter drugs may increase risk for gout in some people. These include:

- Diuretics
- Aspirin or other drugs that contain salicylates
- Niacin, a vitamin that is also called nicotinic acid
- Cyclosporine, which is often used to prevent organ rejection after transplantations
- Levodopa, a common drug used to treat Parkinson's disease

Gravel Root Gout Tincture

Use this valuable tincture to alleviate the symptoms of gout.

2 parts gravel root
2 parts couch grass
2 parts celery seed
1 part guaiacum

To make: Combine all ingredients. Make a tincture following the instructions on page 104.
To use: Take 1 teaspoon (5 ml) of the tincture 3 times per day.

Lifestyle Treatments

Gout appears to be common among people who have diets that include meat and animal fats, but it is unusual in people who follow vegetarian diets. Here are some other lifestyle guidelines for preventing attacks of gout:

- Avoid purine-rich foods, including anchovies, asparagus, crab, fish roe (eggs), herring, kidney meats, liver meats, sweetbreads, meat-based gravies and broths, mushrooms, mussels, peas, beans, and sardines.
- Avoid diets that promote rapid weight loss. Dropping pounds too quickly may result in increased uric acid levels in the blood.
- Avoid all alcoholic drinks.
- Drink 6 pints of fluid a day. Slightly alkaline natural spring water is recommended. This helps dilute the urine and promotes excretion of uric acid.
- Eat raw fruit, vegetables, grains, seeds, and nuts.

- Eat ½ pound fresh or canned cherries a day. Cherries help lower uric acid levels. Along with hawthorn berries, blueberries, and other dark red-blue berries, they are rich sources of anthocyanidins and proanthocyanidins. These compounds help prevent the breakdown of collagen during gouty inflammation by reinforcing the collagen matrix of connective tissue and minimizing free radical damage.
- Exercise regularly and maintain a healthy body weight. Lose weight if you are overweight.

To quickly relieve pain during an acute attack, fill a plastic bag with ice or take a bag of frozen vegetables, wrap the bag in a towel, and apply the pack to the tender area for up to 5 minutes at a time. Cold will help numb the pain and reduce swelling. Keep in mind, however, that the pain of gout can be so tremendous that you may be unable to put pressure on the affected area. Since even the pressure of a sheet or blanket can be painful during a gout attack, at bedtime you may want to place your foot in a cardboard box, or in a plastic laundry basket turned on its side.

MYALGIA ("RHEUMATISM")

Rheumatism is a notoriously vague and often misused description for various muscle aches and pains. However, rheumatic pains are often an early sign of infection and a variety of autoimmune conditions; careful diagnosis is necessary. Since this type of diagnosis is often beyond the expertise of an herbalist, if the symptoms can't be eased within 2 weeks you should seek the help of a physician.

Treating with Herbs

Most of the salicylate-containing anti-inflammatories are considered specific in the various folk traditions of the world. Especially important are meadowsweet, wintergreen, white poplar, and willow bark. In addition, all other antirheumatics — particularly angelica and celery seed — can be used. External applications of rubefacients, salicin-containing oils, circulatory stimulants, or even antispasmodics will often help. It all depends on what the patient best responds to.

The musculoskeletal system as a whole also needs support in the form of tonics. For example:

- If the discomfort is due to a long-standing sports injury, the connective tissue must be strengthened with the appropriate tonic. At the same time, an antispasmodic will be needed to relax the muscles.
- If you have a history of digestive problems, digestive tonics are indicated.
- If you have hypertension or heart disease, use cardiovascular tonics. The herbs and lifestyle treatments to be combined for this type of condition should be left up to the professional judgment of an herbalist.

Remember that long-term stress can lead to tense muscles, which may, in turn, bind the joints too tightly. The resulting friction can develop into wear-and-tear arthritis (osteoarthritis) and in the short term will cause pain and stiffness.

Rheumatism Tincture

Included here is a basic range of antirheumatics that contain salicylates and have anti-inflammatory action. This formula also supports the digestive process and acts as a general alterative.

> 1 part willow bark
> 1 part meadowsweet
> 1 part nettle

To make: Combine all ingredients. Make a tincture following the directions on page 104.
To use: Take 1 teaspoon (5 ml) of the tincture 3 times per day.

TOPICAL RELIEF

External applications of many kinds can help relieve the discomfort of myalgia. These herbal applications may be antispasmodic, rubefacient, or anti-inflammatory in nature. Below is a listing of several valuable topical herbs.

- **Bay tree** *(Laurus nobilis)* oil is good for an assortment of rheumatic and arthritic aches and pains.

- **Black mustard** *(Brassica nigra)* seeds, used in a poultice, can help ease local pain, sciatica, and gout. Mix the powdered seeds with warm water to form a paste. Spread the paste on brown paper and apply it to the affected area. Mustard oil, a powerful local irritant, may be incorporated into liniments for rheumatic pain.

- **Cayenne** *(Capsicum* spp.) stimulates local circulation, making it a good choice for arthritis and rheumatism. Mix 1 part cayenne with ½ part mullein leaf and ½ part slippery elm, and add apple cider vinegar to moisten the mixture. If it burns too much, apply vegetable oil to the skin before using the poultice. In addition, equal parts cayenne and glycerin can be mixed together, then applied to painful joints. Cayenne powder or tincture can also be rubbed on swelling and inflammations for added relief.

- **Lavender** *(Lavandula officinalis)* essential oil, when added in small amounts to a fixed oil such as almond, makes a very useful anti-inflammatory for most rheumatic conditions.

- **Mullein** *(Verbascum thapsus)* combines well with black cohosh and lobelia to make a liniment. Or use mullein infused oil by itself; either rub the oil directly into the skin, or saturate a cloth with it and apply the cloth to the affected area.

- **White mustard** *(Brassica alba)* seeds mixed with black mustard seeds, mustard flowers, bread crumbs, and vinegar can be used in poultices for rheumatic and sciatic pains. Although the treatment may redden the skin, it is very stimulating and efficient.

Lobelia–Cramp Bark Antispasmodic

This external treatment is a nice accompaniment to the internal tincture described below.

> 1 part lobelia
> 1 part cramp bark

To make: Combine the ingredients. Make a tincture following the instructions on page 104.
To use: Apply the tincture externally to sore muscles as needed.

Antispasmodic Treatment

For the relief of muscle cramps or other rheumatic aches and pains, try this tincture.

> 1 part lobelia, powdered
> 1 part skunk cabbage
> 1 part skullcap
> 1 part gum myrrh
> 1 part valerian
> ½ part cayenne

To make: Combine all ingredients. Make a tincture following the instructions on page 104; use brandy as the menstruum. Infuse in a covered container for 1 week, shaking daily. Strain and press out the clear liquid.
To use: Apply to affected areas as needed.

Liniment for Rheumatic Problems

This traditional North American liniment will ease many types of rheumatic discomfort.

> 1 part sassafras tincture
> 1 part prickly ash tincture
> 1 part cayenne tincture
> 1 part myrrh tincture
> 1 part camphor tincture
> 8 parts distilled water

To make: Combine all ingredients in a bottle. Shake well.
To use: Apply to affected areas as needed.

OSTEOARTHRITIS

Also called "wear-and-tear" arthritis or degenerative joint disease, osteoarthritis is the most common form of this condition. It affects about one in six Americans, including 80 percent of those 70 and older. Both men and women can get osteoarthritis, although they tend to develop it at different times. Among men, it's more common for those under age 45; for women, it's more common after age 45.

To understand osteoarthritis, it helps to know how the joints are constructed. Joints, places where two moving bones come together, are designed to protect the bone ends from wearing away and to absorb shock from movements, such as walking or typing. Joints contain the following parts:

- **Cartilage.** A hard but slippery coating on the ends of each bone, cartilage is broken down and worn away in osteoarthritis.

- **Joint capsule.** This tough membrane sac holds the bones and other joint parts together.
- **Synovium.** This is a thin membrane inside the joint capsule.
- **Synovial fluid.** A liquid lubricant that helps the joint move smoothly and also keeps the cartilage smooth and healthy.
- **Muscles, ligaments, and tendons.** Muscles are the tissues that control body movement. Ligaments are tough, cordlike tissues that connect one bone to another. Tendons are tough, fibrous cords that connect muscles to bones. Together, these tissues keep bones stable and allow joints to bend and move.

Osteoarthritis mostly affects the cartilage of the joints. Healthy cartilage allows bones to glide over one another while reducing jolts and shocks. In people with osteoarthritis, the surface layer of the cartilage breaks down and wears away. This allows bones to rub against each other, resulting in pain, swelling, and a reduction of motion in the joint. Bone spurs — the bony equivalent of scar tissue — may form, further impeding normal motion. Sometimes bits of bone or cartilage break off and float inside the joint space, causing more pain and damage. Over time, the joint may lose its normal shape.

Unlike other forms of arthritis, osteoarthritis affects only the joints. It doesn't harm the internal organs the way rheumatoid arthritis might. Although osteoarthritis can occur in any joint, it usually affects the following:

- **Hands.** Small, bony knobs (known as Heberden's nodes) may appear on the distal interphalangeal joints, the end joints of the fingers. Similar knobs may appear on the middle joints. The fingers can become enlarged and gnarled, and they often ache, stiffen, or turn numb. The base of the thumb joint is often affected.
- **Knees.** These are the body's primary weight-bearing joints. They are commonly affected by osteoarthritis, becoming stiff, swollen, and painful.

Bogbean–Meadowsweet Tincture

This remedy combines antirheumatics that have a range of other relevant actions. Note: Devil's claw may be used in place of bogbean, and willow can be substituted for meadowsweet.

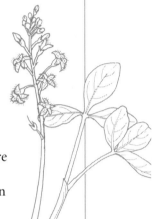

2 parts bogbean
1½ parts meadowsweet
1 part black cohosh
1 part prickly ash
1 part celery seed
1 part angelica
1 part yarrow

To make: Combine all ingredients. Make a tincture following the instructions on page 104.
To use: Take 1 teaspoon (5 ml) of the combination tincture 3 times per day.

Insomnia Remedy

Osteoarthritis can make sleeping difficult. It's necessary to do something about this because much healing happens during sleep.

1 part Jamaican dogwood
1 part kava kava
1 part passionflower

To make: Combine all ingredients. Make a tincture following the instructions on page 104.
To use: Take 1 teaspoon (5 ml) of the combination tincture 30 minutes before going to bed. It's safe to take a stronger dose — up to 2 teaspoons (10 ml) — if required.

- **Hips.** Osteoarthritis in the hips can cause severe disability. The pain may be felt not only in the hips but also in the groin, inner thighs, or knees. Even simple daily activities can become a challenge.
- **Spine.** Stiffness may occur in the neck or lower back. In some cases, the arms and legs will also become numb or weak.

Treating with Herbs

Antirheumatics usually help, but your selection should be based on sound therapeutic rationale; read up on the plants you think might be best for your condition, taking into consideration any other health conditions as well as your lifestyle. Bogbean is an excellent choice for most people.

Anti-inflammatories relieve discomfort and also help stop degenerative changes. Especially helpful are salicylate-based herbs, such as meadowsweet.

Alteratives are the key to correcting systemic problems, if such problems are present. Bogbean is primary for osteoarthritis.

Antispasmodics lessen the effect of physical friction by relaxing the muscles that surround the joints. Black cohosh proves effective here.

Circulatory stimulants benefit the healing process by increasing the flow of blood. The bark or berries of prickly ash is helpful. Bogbean and devil's claw could be considered specifics for osteoarthritis. However, you must also keep in mind that a single herbal action is not always the key to healing; the whole plant offers many different benefits. Nettle is a traditional remedy throughout Europe, where it is used internally and externally as a rubefacient. The external use, in which the fresh "stinging nettle" leaf is applied to the skin, is not for the fainthearted. During a recent study at Plymouth Medical School in Great Britain researchers noted, "No observed side effects were reported, except a transient urticarial rash"!

> ## THE WARNING SIGNS OF OSTEOARTHRITIS
>
> It usually takes years for osteoarthritis to start producing serious symptoms. The warning signs include:
>
> - Steady or intermittent pain in a joint.
> - Stiffness after getting out of bed.
> - Swelling or tenderness in one or more joints.
> - A "crunching" feeling as bone rubs on bone.
>
> Warmth, redness, and tenderness are generally not signs of osteoarthritis. Keep in mind, also, that not everyone with osteoarthritis feels pain. Only one-third of patients whose osteoarthritis has been discovered on X-rays report pain or other symptoms.

External Remedies for Osteoarthritis

Ointments and other topical remedies can ease pain and reduce inflammation while at the same time stimulating circulation to the affected area. The enhanced circulation helps eliminate pain-causing toxins that may be contributing to the damage. While such a treatment will not by itself cause fundamental change, it will facilitate the healing process and lessen discomfort. To make a simple liniment that's both warming and stimulating, mix equal parts of glycerine and tincture of cayenne. Rub the liniment into the affected joints or muscles. Don't use the liniment on broken skin or facial skin, however; it's not harmful, but it may cause a burning sensation for a short time. This same heat relieves pain in cold, aching joints and stiff muscles.

Lifestyle Treatments

Herbal treatments by themselves aren't enough to stop the pain and degeneration caused by osteoarthritis. This condition truly requires a multifaceted approach.

St.-John's-Wort Healing Liniment

If you're experiencing pain in muscle tissue or any type of nerve pain, a liniment that includes St.-John's-wort oil can be effective. Make the liniment in late summer, when the herb blossoms have just opened.

- 4 ounces (100 g) fresh, just-opened St.-John's-wort blossoms
- 1 pint (400 ml) plus 1 tablespoon (15 ml) olive or sunflower oil

To make:
1. Crush the blossoms in the tablespoon of olive or sunflower oil. Place the mixture in a clear glass container.
2. Cover the mixture with the pint of olive or sunflower oil. Mix well.
3. Store the open container in a warm place to ferment for 3–5 days. Next, seal the container well and place it in sunshine or another warm place for 3–6 weeks, shaking daily, until the oil is bright red.
4. Strain out the plant material by pressing the mixture through a cloth suspended over a bowl or bottle. Let the oil stand for a day until it separates from the watery part of the mixture.
5. Strain out the watery part and discard. Store the oil in an opaque, air-tight container.

To use: Rub the liniment on the affected areas as needed. This remedy can also be used on mild burns.

Exercise is essential for improving mood and outlook, decreasing pain, increasing flexibility, improving blood flow, maintaining weight, and promoting general physical fitness. However, the amount and form of exercise depend on which joints are involved, how stable they are, and whether a joint replacement has been done. Talk to your doctor or physical therapist about setting up an exercise program that's right for you. The following types of exercise will most likely be indicated:

- **Strength.** Exercise bands are inexpensive devices that can be used to build strength through resistance.
- **Aerobic.** Activities that keep your lungs and circulatory system in shape will enhance stamina and encourage toxin elimination.
- **Range of motion.** These exercises are used to keep the joints limber.
- **Agility.** Many people find that their "daily living" skills are improved with agility exercises.
- **Neck and back strength.** In addition to performing regular strength exercises, participate in activities aimed at keeping your spine strong and limber.

Consult your physician or physical therapist to determine which exercise program is appropriate for your condition.

Rest is critical. It is important to recognize the body's signals and to know when to stop or slow down. People who overexercise or push themselves too hard will experience more pain and joint damage.

Special joint care also requires attention. Some people find that relaxation, stress reduction, and biofeedback techniques work well. But your doctor may recommend using a cane or a splint to restrict joint movement and reduce pressure. Although splints provide extra support for weakened joints, they must be used only for limited periods; joints and muscles need to be exercised in order to prevent stiffness and weakness.

Pain relief therapies will make you feel better, at least temporarily. As we've discussed, there are many nonpharmaceutical methods for relieving osteoarthritis pain. Warm towels, hot packs, or warm baths apply moist heat to the joint, alleviating pain and stiffness. In some cases, especially acute inflammation, cold packs (such as a bag of ice or frozen vegetables wrapped in a towel) can reduce pain in the sore area. Water therapy in a heated pool may also relieve pain and stiffness.

Weight control is all-important because a lower body weight will further reduce stress on weight-bearing joints and limit further injury.

If you are becoming disabled because of this disease, consider using physical aids and supports. There is a wealth of simple devices — known as Activities of Daily Living (ADI) devices — that will aid you in the normal daily tasks that have become taxing. Equipment ranges from specially designed kitchen tools (such as cutlery, can openers, and faucet grips) to hairbrushes with extended handles and adaptive pieces for telephones. Using these devices can help you enormously. Consult your physical therapist and occupational therapist for more information, or contact the Arthritis Foundation (see Resources) or local organizations dedicated to helping aging people.

Nutritional Factors

Diet can be very important in the treatment of osteoarthritis. There has been a lot of discussion and controversy in recent years about appropriate dietary and supplement therapies. I do not want to enter such confused debates at this stage, but it is appropriate to point out that changes in diet can make a difference.

What you eat may be less important than what you don't eat. Some foods definitely aggravate arthritic problems. Try to avoid the following:

- Coffee, caffeinated or decaffeinated
- Red meat of any kind
- Vinegar and vinegar-based foods, such as pickles (apple cider vinegar may be an exception)
- Vegetables that contain high levels of plant acids, such as tomatoes and rhubarb
- Plants of the nightshade family, including tomatoes, eggplant, peppers, potatoes, and tobacco

- Berries rich in fruit acids, such as gooseberries and red and black currants
- Refined white flour and products that contain it
- Artificial additives, flavorings, and preservatives
- Processed foods
- Red wine, port, and sherry
- Carbonated drinks
- Shellfish
- Any food or beverage that you suspect is exacerbating symptoms

One more note about diet: Avoiding certain foods will produce the best results in the earlier, more painful stages of this drawn-out disease. Obviously, you'll have to find your own balance between the benefits of avoiding certain foods and the psychological benefits that come from eating foods you enjoy.

HELPFUL SUPPLEMENTS

A variety of nutritional supplements may be helpful for people with osteoarthritis. According to *The Textbook of Natural Medicine,* by Drs. Pizzorno and Murray, the following supplements may be worth a try:

- Copper, 1 mg per day
- Glucosamine sulfate, 1500 mg per day
- Methionine, 400 mg 3 times per day
- Pantothenic acid, 12.5 mg per day
- Vitamin A, 5000 IU per day
- Vitamin B_6, 50 mg per day
- Vitamin C, 1000–2000 mg per day
- Vitamin E, 600 IU per day
- Zinc, 45 mg per day

OSTEOPOROSIS

Osteoporosis weakens bones to the point that they break easily. Bones in the hips, spine, and wrist are especially vulnerable. About 25 million Americans, approximately 80 percent of them women, have osteoporosis. One out of two women and one in eight men over the age of 50 will have an osteoporosis-related fracture.

Although the exact cause of osteoporosis is unknown, the process by which the bones become weak, or porous, is understood. In a normal adult, the body replaces 6 to 12 percent of the total skeleton with new bone cells each year. After skeletal mass peaks — usually around age 35 — bones begin to lose calcium (the mineral that makes them hard) faster than they can replace it. For women, this loss of bone density accelerates during the first 3 to 7 years after the onset of menopause and then slows down again.

This postmenopausal increase in bone loss is thought to be caused by the decline of estrogen that accompanies menopause. In addition, several conditions, such as kidney disease, Cushing's syndrome, and hyperthyroidism, reduce the ability of the body to absorb calcium. Surgical removal of part of the stomach or intestine and excessive use of steroids (including glucocorticoids) or anticonvulsant drugs can also have this effect. Prolonged immobility, due to a long illness, for example, can also result in bone loss.

Unlike many bone and joint problems, osteoporosis is preventable. Dietary factors are critical, as is regular exercise.

Calcium and Diet

Calcium is essential for maintaining strong bones. Fortunately, it's possible to get large amounts of calcium in the diet. Calcium-rich foods include:

- Low-fat dairy products, such as cheese, yogurt, and milk
- Canned fish with small, edible bones, such as salmon and sardines

- Dark green leafy vegetables, such as kale, collard, spinach, and broccoli
- Breads made with calcium-fortified flour.

The diets of most people only provide one-third to one-half of the calcium they need. The low intake is especially dangerous for women, who have higher calcium requirement. Calcium supplements can make up the difference. Look for chelated forms of calcium, such as calcium citrate and calcium gluconate, which are more easily absorbed.

Vitamin D is necessary for optimal calcium absorption. The body can produce its own vitamin D simply by being exposed to the sun for short periods every day. But if you don't live in a sunny geographical location or aren't able to get outside very often, you may need vitamin D supplements (400 to 800 IU per day).

Magnesium is another necessity for optimal calcium absorption. The recommended daily dose is 250 to 350 mg.

Phytoestrogens are plant chemicals that resemble estrogens. Herbs containing phytoestrogens have long been used to treat conditions that are now treated with synthetic drugs. These herbs may be suitable alternatives to estrogen therapy in the prevention of osteoporosis in menopausal women. Soy based foods are a particularly good source of phytoestrogens. They also contain soy isoflavonoids, which have been indicated in the prevention of breast cancer.

Treating with Herbs

Herbal therapies alone cannot eliminate osteoporosis. However, they can slow the process when they're combined with other nutritional and lifestyle strategies. Herbalists have traditionally recommended herbs such as horsetail, oat straw, and alfalfa for the long-term treatment of osteoporosis. These herbs have been thought to be effective because of their high calcium content. Actually, they do not have particularly high levels of calcium, but they are often effective anyway!

WHAT TO AVOID

While it's extremely important to increase your intake of the foods mentioned above, it's also important to avoid phosphorus-rich foods, which can promote bone loss. High-phosphorus foods include:

• Red meats

• Soft drinks

• Foods with phosphate food additives (look for references to phosphate or phosphoric acid in the ingredient lists)

Excessive amounts of alcohol and caffeine are thought to reduce the amount of calcium absorbed by the body. These substances should be avoided or taken in moderation.

Chasteberry Remedy

Herbal remedies that help normalize the body's hormones may be helpful if they're started early enough. In addition, anti-rheumatics will ease pain that may occur in the joints or muscles. Take this remedy in either tincture or tea form.

> 2 parts chasteberry
> 1 part horsetail
> 1 part oats
> 1 part alfalfa

To make: Combine all ingredients. If making a tincture, follow the instructions on page 104. If making an infusion, follow the instructions on page 102 (infuse for 20 minutes).
To use: Take 1 teaspoon (5 ml) of the tincture or 1 cup (240 ml) of the infusion 3 times per day.

Preventing Osteoporosis

Because osteoporosis is preventable, you can take several steps to protect your bones. Here are some important basic guidelines:

- Eat foods rich in calcium, such as low-fat milk, low-fat yogurt, broccoli, cauliflower, salmon, tofu, sesame seeds, almonds, and leafy green vegetables.
- If you are a woman, eat foods that contain plant estrogens, especially tofu and other soy products.
- Avoid foods that can interfere with your body's absorption of calcium, such as red meats, soft drinks, and excessive amounts of alcohol and caffeine.
- Do weight-bearing exercises, which put some stress on the bones, for 30 to 45 minutes at least 3 times per week. Regular exercise not only increases bone strength but also helps prevent bone loss. Weight-bearing exercises include dancing, running, walking, stair-climbing, and aerobics.
- Don't smoke. This unhealthy activity is associated with lowered bone mineral density in both sexes. Some studies have shown that women who smoke increase their risk of developing osteoporosis by 50 percent.
- Avoid antacids that contain aluminum; they can interfere with calcium absorption by binding with phosphorus in the intestines.

RESTLESS LEG SYNDROME

This syndrome is a puzzling neurological disorder for which there is presently no cure. The condition is characterized by a tingling or crawling sensation deep in the legs, which causes an overwhelming need to move the legs to relieve the discomfort. Symptoms often worsen at night.

Restless leg syndrome is believed to be brought on by a chemical imbalance in the brain, and it also appears to be genetic. The

A LIFETIME OF CALCIUM

At the 1994 Consensus Development Conference on Optimal Calcium Intake, a panel convened by the National Institutes of Health determined the optimal amounts of calcium that people need to ingest daily at different ages and stages of their lives.

- Birth–6 months: 400 mg
- 6–12 months: 600 mg
- 1–5 years: 800 mg
- 6–10 years: 800–1200 mg
- 11–24 years: 1200–1500 mg
- Women between 25 and 50 years: 1000 mg
- Women who are pregnant or lactating: 1200–1500 mg
- Postmenopausal women using estrogen replacement therapy: 1000 mg
- Postmenopausal women not using estrogen therapy: 1500 mg
- Men between 25 and 65 years: 1000 mg
- All women and men over 65 years: 1500 mg

condition has also been linked to iron or folic acid deficiencies, especially in people with kidney disease. Research shows that caffeine can increase symptoms.

Treating with Herbs

Herbs with strong relaxing qualities may be effective in reducing muscle tension and relieving pain. These plants include:

- Passionflower
- Valerian
- Kava kava
- Black cohosh

In addition, cramp bark often helps relax muscles.

Although there is no cure for restless leg syndrome, these steps can reduce the frequency and intensity of symptoms:

- Take a multivitamin with iron, as well as vitamin E and a B-complex supplement to help correct the nutrient deficiencies that may contribute to symptoms.
- Take 400 to 1000 mcg of folic acid to offset any deficiency.
- Avoid stimulants, such as caffeine and decongestants.
- Avoid stimulating activities for up to three hours before bedtime; these include exercising and eating heavy meals.
- Keep the bedroom quiet and cool; an overly warm room may aggravate the condition.
- Practice stress-reduction and relaxation techniques such as yoga, biofeedback, and meditation.
- Soak the feet in cool water; the cooling action may be effective in bringing relief. Never use ice water, however, because it can cause nerve damage.

TRY LEG MASSAGE

This treatment can help relieve the symptoms of restless leg syndrome.

1. Sit on the floor and bend one knee; keep the foot flat. Grasp your calf with both hands and use your thumbs to find the muscle that runs along the outside of the shinbone, below the kneecap. Massage the muscle all the way down to the anklebone.

2. Place both thumbs on the inside of the leg near the anklebone. Keeping the hands around the calf for support, massage the inside of the leg vigorously with both thumbs. Massage from the ankle up to the knee.

3. Use the thumbs and other fingers of both hands to knead the back and sides of the calf muscle. Work from the knee down to the ankle. Repeat all steps on the other leg. Alternate massaging both legs several times.

RHEUMATOID ARTHRITIS

More than two million Americans have rheumatoid arthritis, a chronic inflammatory condition that involves not only the joints but also other connective tissue. The disease is found in all ethnic groups and often begins in middle age and occurs with increased frequency in older people. However, children and young adults also develop it. Like some other forms of arthritis, rheumatoid arthritis is seen much more often in women than in men. Although we don't understand why, about two to three times as many women as men have it.

Rheumatoid arthritis is one of several autoimmune diseases; it occurs when the immune system attacks the body's own tissues. No one knows exactly what causes this phenomenon. An important laboratory finding is the presence of rheumatoid factor (RF) in people with rheumatoid arthritis. RF is a special antibody that attacks the normal antibodies in the bloodstream. The reasons RF develops are unknown, but researchers suspect that it is caused by an exaggerated immune response to long-term stimulation by infectious agents or other foreign substances. Rheumatoid factor itself is not directly responsible for the inflammatory process; it acts solely as a marker for the disease.

The joint destruction that occurs with severe rheumatoid arthritis results from inflammation of the synovia, the thin, smooth membranes or capsules lining the joints. White blood cells and antibodies infiltrate the synovial membranes, causing the membranes to proliferate and fold over on themselves. Persistent or recurrent inflammation causes permanent damage to the joint cartilage, bones, ligaments, and tendons. The widespread inflammatory process also involves other tissues, such as blood vessels, skin, nerves, muscles, and the heart and lungs. The result is painful joints, loss of mobility, and generalized soreness and depression.

For about 5 to 10 percent of people with rheumatoid arthritis, the condition is mild or limited to one or two episodes. About 25 percent of people have an erratic pattern of prolonged remissions and periods of relapse. For most people, however, the disease never goes away entirely, and flare-ups occur intermittently.

Most people continue to function despite some pain and discomfort. However, about 10 percent of those with rheumatoid arthritis have permanent joint damage and serious limitation of movement.

Although the symptoms of rheumatoid arthritis vary, pain, swelling, stiffness, and loss of function in the joints are usually observed. Sometimes fatigue, occasional fever, and a general sense of malaise occur. Unlike other forms of arthritis, rheumatoid arthritis generally occurs symmetrically; if, for instance, one hand develops symptoms, the other will too.

This disease often affects the wrist joints and finger joints that are closest to the hand, but other non-joint parts of the body can be affected. Rheumatoid arthritis may last only a few months and then go away without causing any noticeable damage. It may take the form of a mild or moderate disease, with periods of worsening symptoms (flares) followed by periods in which people feel better (remissions). The severe form of rheumatoid arthritis is active most of the time, lasts for many years, and leads to serious joint damage and disability.

Treating with Herbs

Antirheumatics usually help (as is the case with osteoarthritis), but their use should be determined based on the individual. Bogbean is a frequent choice of antirheumatic.

Anti-inflammatories are very important because most symptoms of rheumatoid arthritis involve painful inflammation. Anti-inflammatories containing phytosterols, such as wild yam and bupleurum, come into their own here. However, the salicylate herbs are still helpful, and meadowsweet is an excellent choice. These two classes of herbs complement each other well.

THE WARNING SIGNS OF RHEUMATOID ARTHRITIS

Since rheumatoid arthritis can be an extremely serious condition, it's essential to be alert to the warning signs. These include:

• Joint pain and stiffness that come on gradually.

• An initial period of pain followed by joint swelling, redness, and warmth, usually within a few weeks.

• Symptoms developing in the hands, wrists, shoulders, elbows, feet, ankles, and knees on both sides of the body. In some cases, inflammation of a single joint may be the first sign.

• Symptoms that are severe in the morning and diminish later on with movement.

• Small, firm lumps called rheumatoid nodules can be felt beneath the skin, especially around the elbow.

• Fatigue in the early afternoon and difficulty sleeping at night.

Be aware that rheumatoid arthritis can also affect other organs. Vasculitis, an inflammation of the blood vessels, can cause skin rashes, ulcers, and gangrene. Other manifestations including scarring of the lungs, inflammation of the membranes surrounding the heart and lungs, nerve damage, dry eyes and mouth (Sjögrens syndrome), and enlargement of the spleen and lymph nodes.

Alteratives play a pivotal role in any immune system illness. Although we do not know its exact mechanism of action, bogbean is an essential herbal alterative.

Antispasmodics, such as black cohosh, relieve muscular tension caused by pain and stress.

Circulatory stimulants are less important for rheumatoid arthritis than for osteoarthritis. Similarly, the rubefacients aren't necessary and can in fact worsen symptoms.

Hypnotics encourage sleep; this is an especially important concern in conditions that are chronically painful.

Nervines are especially helpful because of the psychosomatic nature of this problem. Nervine relaxants will ease spasms, while nervine tonics help the person deal with the constant stress from the pain and discomfort.

Tonics and antidepressants help people cope with this very tiring and debilitating condition.

Eight-Herb Tincture for Rheumatoid Arthritis

There are no specific remedies for rheumatoid arthritis; it is a complex disease with a multitude of immunological factors. But alterative-based antirheumatics are particularly relevant — including bogbean, devil's claw, and burdock. Guaiacum, meadowsweet, bupleurum, black cohosh, and wild yam are all effective anti-inflammatories. Also included are antispasmodics (black cohosh and celery seed), a nervine tonic/antidepressant (St.-John's-wort), a diuretic (celery seed), and carminatives (meadowsweet and celery seed).

2 parts bogbean
2 parts meadowsweet
1 part wild yam
1 part guaiacum
1 part black cohosh
1 part celery seed
1 part bupleurum
1 part St.-John's-wort

To make: Combine all ingredients. Make a tincture following the instructions on page 104.
To use: Take 1 teaspoon (5 ml) of the tincture 3 times per day.

Insomnia Reliever

As in osteoarthritis, the pain of rheumatoid arthritis can make it difficult for you to sleep. If you are suffering from insomnia, try this simple tincture.

> 1 part valerian
> 1 part Jamaican dogwood
> 1 part passionflower

To make: Combine all ingredients. Make a tincture following the instructions on page 104.
To use: Take 1–3 teaspoon (5–15 ml) of the tincture 30 minutes before going to bed.

Lifestyle Treatments

The dietary advice given for osteoarthritis, discussed on page 51, is equally pertinent here. You may also want to try supplements; see the box on the following page for more information.

You need to achieve a good balance between rest and exercise, with more rest when the disease is active and more exercise when it is not. Rest helps reduce active joint inflammation and pain and eases fatigue. Shorter rest breaks every now and then are more helpful than longer ones. Exercise, on the other hand, maintains healthy and strong muscles, preserves joint mobility, and improves flexibility. Physical activity can also promote sleep, reduce pain, help you lose weight, and encourage a positive attitude.

Rheumatoid arthritis is often as much of an emotional challenge as a physical one. The emotions commonly experienced with this condition — fear, anger, frustration — can greatly increase the person's level of stress. Although stress probably does not cause rheumatoid arthritis, it makes coping with the disease much more difficult. Fortunately, there are a number of effective techniques for coping with stress, including regular rest and relaxation, distraction, or visualization exercises.

HELPFUL SUPPLEMENTS

These supplements have been recommended by Drs. Pizzorno and Murray in *The Textbook of Natural Medicine* for the treatment of rheumatoid arthritis:

- Copper, 1 mg per day
- DHEA (dehydroepiandrosterone sulfate), 50–200 mg per day
- EPA (eicosapentaenoic acid), 1.8 g per day; or flaxseed oil, 1 tablespoon (15 ml) per day
- Manganese, 15 mg per day
- Pantothenic acid, 500 mg four times per day
- Selenium, 200 micrograms per day
- Quercetin, 250 mg between meals 3 times per day
- Vitamin C, 1000–3000 mg per day
- Vitamin E, 400 IU per day
- Zinc, 45 mg per day

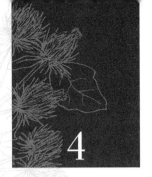

A GUIDE
TO THE HEALING HERBS

Herbs have been used for centuries to treat a wide variety of ailments. Although herbs have been largely disregarded by allopathic medicine, researchers are now rediscovering what herbalists have known all along: Phytotherapy, or treatment with plants, affords us more versatility with far less adverse reactions than do chemical drugs.

The green world offers us a veritable cornucopia of healing herbs. Careful selection from this rich abundance can provide a range of safe, effective, and pleasant healing agents for both maintaining the health of the musculoskeletal system and treating many of its maladies.

The herbs described in this section are those most likely to be of help for the conditions described in this book. They have been selected for their efficacy, ease of use, and availability. Remember that herbs generally don't have one specific action; they are composed of a variety of complex constituents that have a multifaceted effect on the body. Thus, when choosing herbs to treat a musculoskeletal condition, also consider any other systems that might need support. In this way, you will not only treat the specific problem but also any other areas that require help.

ANGELICA *(Angelica archangelica)*

Parts Used: Roots and leaves

Actions: Anti-inflammatory, astringent, cholagogue, diuretic, tonic, vulnerary

Indications: Angelica herb is a useful expectorant for coughs, bronchitis, and pleurisy, especially when they are accompanied by fever, colds, or influenza. The leaf can be used as a compress for inflammations of the chest. It contains a carminative essential oil, making it useful for intestinal colic and flatulence. As a digestive, it stimulates appetite and may be used in anorexia nervosa. It has been shown to help ease rheumatic inflammations. For cystitis, it acts as a urinary antiseptic.

Angelica is used frequently as a flavoring, such as in the liqueurs chartreuse and benedictine, as well as in gin and vermouth. The leaves can be used as a garnish or in salads, and the candied stalks are a nice addition to cakes and puddings.

Preparations and Dosage: To make a decoction, put 1 teaspoon cut root in 1 cup water. Bring to a boil, then simmer 2 minutes. Remove from heat and let stand 15 minutes. Take 1 cup 3 times per day.

As a tincture, take 2–5 ml 3 times per day.

ARNICA *(Arnica montana)*

Part Used: Flower heads

Actions: Anti-inflammatory, vulnerary

Indications: This herb is considered toxic and should not be taken internally. (However, the homeopathic preparation is entirely safe to take internally.) It is one of the best remedies for external local healing and is often recommended for bruises and sprains.

Arnica helps relieve rheumatic pain as well as the pain and inflammation of phlebitis and similar conditions. It is also considered an immuno-stimulant.

Preparation and Dosage: You can prepare a tincture of arnica as follows: In a clear glass container, pour 1 pint (½ liter) 70 percent alcohol over 2 ounces (50 g) freshly picked flowers. Seal the container tightly and let it stand for at least a week in the sun or other warm place. Strain and rebottle. Rub into the affected areas as needed.

Caution: This herb is toxic and should *not* be taken internally. Do not use externally on broken skin.

Balm of Gilead (*Populus* x *jackii* 'Gileadensis')

Part Used: Closed buds

Actions: Antimicrobial, stimulating expectorant, vulnerary

Indications: Balm of Gilead soothes, disinfects, and acts as an astringent on the mucous membranes; this makes it an excellent remedy for sore throats, coughs, and laryngitis. It is considered to be a specific for laryngitis that is accompanied by voice loss. It may be used in chronic bronchitis. Externally, it can be used to ease inflammations due to rheumatism and arthritis and to treat dry and scaly skin conditions, such as psoriasis and dry eczema.

Preparations and Dosage: To make an infusion, pour 1 cup boiling water over 1 teaspoon buds; steep 10–15 minutes. Drink 3 times per day or more often — if you can stand the taste!

As a tincture, take 1–2 ml 3 times per day.

BAYBERRY *(Myrica cerifera)*

Part Used: Root

Actions: Astringent, circulatory stimulant, diaphoretic

Indications: Bayberry is widely used as a circulatory stimulant. As a specific, it's a valuable astringent for diarrhea and dysentery. It may be used for mucous colitis. As a gargle, it helps sore throats. As a douche, this herb is helpful for people with leukorrhea. It may also be used in the treatment of colds.

Preparations and Dosage: To make a decoction, put 1 teaspoon root in 1 cup cold water. Bring to a boil, then simmer 10–15 minutes. Drink 3 times per day.

As a tincture, take 1–2 ml 3 times per day.

BEARBERRY *(Arctostaphylos uva-ursi)*

Part Used: Leaves

Actions: Antimicrobial, astringent, demulcent, diuretic

Indications: Bearberry has a specific antiseptic and astringent effect on the membranes of the urinary system, helping to soothe, tone, and strengthen them. It is specifically used when there is gravel or ulceration in the kidney or bladder. It may be used in the treatment of infections such as pyelitis and cystitis, or as part of a holistic approach to chronic kidney problems. With its high astringency, it is useful for some forms of bedwetting. As a douche, it may be helpful in vaginal ulceration and infection.

Preparations and Dosage: To make an infusion, pour 1 cup boiling water over 1–2 teaspoons dried herb; steep 10–15 minutes. Drink 3 times per day.

As a tincture, take 2–4 ml 3 times per day.

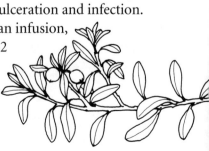

BIRCH (*Betula alba*)

Parts Used: Young leaves and bark
Actions: Anti-inflammatory, antiseptic, diuretic, tonic
Indications: Birch leaves are an effective remedy for cystitis and other infections of the urinary system. They also help remove excess water from the body. Perhaps because of this cleansing, diuretic activity, birch has been used for gout, rheumatism, and mild arthritic pain. The bark will ease muscle pain if it is applied externally: Put the fresh, wet, internal side of the bark against the skin.
Preparations and Dosage: To make an infusion, pour 1 cup boiling water over 1–2 teaspoons dried herb; steep 10 minutes. Drink 3 times per day.

As a tincture, take 1–2 ml 3 times per day.

BLACK COHOSH (*Cimicifuga racemosa*)

Parts Used: Root and rhizome (dried, not fresh)
Actions: Alterative, antispasmodic, emmenagogue, hypotensive, nervine
Indications: Black cohosh is a most valuable herb. It has a powerful action as a relaxant, helps normalize the female reproductive system, and may be used for painful or delayed menstruation. It also relieves ovarian cramps or cramping pain in the womb. It is very active in the treatment of rheumatic pains, rheumatoid arthritis, osteoarthritis, and muscular and neurologic pain. Black cohosh is sometimes used for sciatica and neuralgia. It works as a relaxing nervine and has been found to be beneficial in the treatment of tinnitus.

Few remedies have acquired as great a reputation in the treatment of rheumatism and neuralgia. Indeed, few cases of rheumatism or related conditions are not improved by the use of this herb. Preparations of *Cimicifuga,* to be of any medicinal value, must be prepared from recently dried roots.

Preparations and Dosage: To make a decoction, pour 1 cup water over ½–1 teaspoon dried root. Bring to a boil, then simmer 10–15 minutes. Drink 3 times per day.

As a tincture, take 2–4 ml 3 times per day.

VERSATILE BLACK COHOSH

Kings American Dispensatory, an important textbook of medical herbalism from 1900, included this description of black cohosh:

"This is a very active, powerful, and useful remedy, and appears to fulfill a great number of indications. It possesses an undoubted influence over the nervous system. In small doses the appetite and digestion are improved, and larger amounts augment the secretions of the gastrointestinal tract. Excretions from the skin and kidneys are increased by it, the peculiar earthy odor of the drug being imparted to the urine; the secretions of the bronchial mucous surfaces are also augmented under its administration. The heart-beat is slowed and given increased power by it, while arterial tension is elevated."

⊕BLACK HAW *(Viburnum prunifolium)*

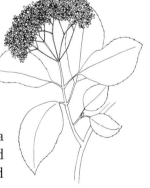

Parts Used: Dried bark of root, stem, or trunk

Actions: Antispasmodic, astringent, hypotensive, nervine

Indications: Black haw is closely related to cramp bark and has similar uses. It is a powerful relaxant of the uterus and is used for dysmenorrhea, false labor pains, and threatened miscarriage. Its relaxant and sedative actions explain its power in reducing blood pressure in hypertension, which it does by relaxing the peripheral blood vessels. It may be used as an antispasmodic in the treatment of asthma.

Preparations and Dosage: To make a decoction, put 2 teaspoons dried bark in 1 cup water. Bring to a boil, then simmer 10 minutes. Drink 3 times per day.

As a tincture, take 5–10 ml 3 times per day.

BOGBEAN *(Menyanthes trifoliata)*

Part Used: Leaves

Actions: Antirheumatic, bitter, cholagogue, diuretic

Indications: Bogbean is a most useful herb for the treatment of rheumatism, osteoarthritis, and rheumatoid arthritis. It has a stimulating effect on the walls of the colon and therefore acts as a laxative, but it should not be used for rheumatism accompanied by colitis or diarrhea. It has a marked stimulating action on the digestive juices and the flow of bile, making it helpful for conditions caused by sluggish digestion, indigestion, or problems with the liver and gallbladder.

Preparations and Dosage: To make an infusion, pour 1 cup boiling water over 1–2 teaspoons dried herb; steep 10–15 minutes. Drink 3 times per day.

As a tincture, take 1–4 ml 3 times per day.

BONESET *(Eupatorium perfoliatum)*

Parts Used: Dried leaves and flowers

Actions: Antispasmodic, astringent, bitter, carminative, diaphoretic, laxative, tonic

Indications: Boneset is one the best remedies for flu symptoms. It speedily relieves the aches and pains and helps the body deal with any fever that may be present. It can also be used to help clear the upper respiratory tract of mucus congestion. Boneset's mild laxative activity eases constipation. It may safely be used for fever and as a general cleansing agent. It may alleviate symptoms of muscular rheumatism.

Preparations and Dosage: To make an infusion, pour 1 cup boiling water over 1–2 teaspoons dried herb; steep 10–15 minutes. This infusion should be drunk as hot as possible. During fevers and flu, drink every 30 minutes until symptoms subside.

As a tincture, take 2–4 ml 3 times per day.

BURDOCK *(Arctium lappa)*

Part Used: Roots and rhizome
Actions: Alterative, bitter, diuretic
Indications: Burdock is a valuable remedy for skin conditions that cause dryness and scaling. It may be effective for psoriasis when used for a long time. As part of a broader treatment plan, it can be used for rheumatic symptoms, especially those associated with psoriasis. Part of the action of burdock occurs through the bitter stimulation of the digestive juices, particularly the stimulation of bile secretion. Thus, it aids digestion and appetite. Burdock has been used in anorexia nervosa and similar conditions. It helps with kidney function and healing of cystitis. In general, this herb moves the body to a state of integration and health.

Externally, it may be used as a compress or poultice to speed wound and ulcer healing. Eczema and psoriasis may also be treated externally. Remember, however, that chronic skin problems can only be healed from within by using internal remedies.

Preparations and Dosage: To make a decoction, put 1 teaspoon root into 1 cup water. Bring to boil, then simmer 10–15 minutes. Drink 3 times per day.

As a tincture, take 2–4 ml 3 times per day.

CALENDULA *(Calendula officinalis)*

Parts Used: Petals, flower heads

Actions: Anti-inflammatory, antimicrobial, antispasmodic, astringent, emmenagogue, lymphatic, vulnerary

Indications: Calendula is one of the best herbs for the treatment of local skin problems, including those caused by infection or physical damage, such as abrasions. It may be used for external bleeding, bruises, strains, slow-healing wounds, and skin ulcers. A lotion or ointment made from this herb is ideal for treating minor burns and scalds, cuts, bruises, diaper rash, and sore nipples. It may also be used in poultices or compresses.

Internally, calendula is a valuable herb for digestive inflammation. It may be used to treat gastric and duodenal ulcers. As a cholagogue, it helps relieve gallbladder problems and indigestion.

Calendula has marked antifungal activity and may be used both internally and externally to combat fungal infections. As an emmenagogue, it has a reputation for helping with delayed menstruation and painful periods.

Preparation and Dosage: To make an infusion, pour 1 cup boiling water over 1–2 teaspoons flowers; steep 10–15 minutes. Drink 3 times per day.

🌿CAYENNE (*Capsicum* spp.)

Part Used: Fruit

Actions: Anticatarrhal, antimicrobial, carminative, rubefacient, sialagogue, stimulant

Indications: Cayenne is the most useful of the systemic stimulants. It stimulates blood flow and strengthens the heart, arteries, capillaries, and nerves. A general tonic, it is specific for both the circulatory and digestive systems. It may be used for flatulent dyspepsia and colic, as well as for cold hands and feet caused by insufficient peripheral circulation. It's also helpful for general debility and for warding off colds.

Externally, cayenne is used as a rubefacient for problems such as lumbago and rheumatic pains. As an ointment, it helps unbroken chilblains, as long as it's used in moderation. As a gargle for laryngitis, it combines well with myrrh. This combination also makes a good antiseptic wash.

Preparations and Dosage: To make an infusion, pour 1 cup boiling water over ½–1 teaspoon dried herb; steep 10 minutes. Mix 1 tablespoon infusion with hot water and drink as needed.

As a tincture, take 0.25–1 ml 3 times per day or as needed.

Caution: May cause eye and skin irritation.

🌿CELERY SEEDS (*Apium graveolens*)

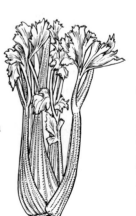

Part Used: Dried ripe fruit

Actions: Anti-inflammatory, antirheumatic, antispasmodic, carminative, diuretic, nervine

Indications: Celery seeds find their main use in the treatment of rheumatism, gout, and arthritis. They are especially useful for rheumatoid arthritis that's accompanied by mental depression.

The diuretic action of this herb not only helps ease rheumatic conditions but is helpful as a urinary antiseptic, largely because of the volatile oil apiol.

Preparations and Dosage: To make an infusion, pour 1 cup boiling water over 1–2 teaspoons freshly crushed seeds. Infuse 10–15 minutes. Drink 3 times per day.

As a tincture, take 1–4 ml 3 times per day.

CLEAVERS *(Galium aparine)*

Parts Used: Dried aerial parts and freshly expressed juice

Actions: Alterative, anti-inflammatory, astringent, diuretic, tonic

Indications: Cleavers is a very valuable plant. It may be the best tonic for the lymphatic system and may be used safely for a wide range of problems affecting that system. These include swollen glands (lymphadenitis) anywhere in the body, especially tonsillitis and adenoid trouble. It is helpful in skin conditions, particularly dry kinds, such as psoriasis. Cleavers can be used to treat cystitis and other urinary conditions accompanied by pain; for this purpose it may be combined with urinary demulcents. The use of cleavers has a long tradition in the treatment of ulcers and tumors. This may be due to its effects on lymphatic drainage, which helps detoxify tissue. Cleavers also makes an excellent vegetable.

Preparations and Dosage: To make an infusion, pour 1 cup boiling water over 2–3 teaspoons dried herb; steep 10–15 minutes. Drink 3 times per day.

As a tincture, take 2–4 ml 3 times per day.

COUCHGRASS *(Elytrigia repens* ssp. *repens)*

Part Used: Rhizome
Actions: Antimicrobial, demulcent, diuretic
Indications: Couchgrass (often called quackgrass in North America) may be used for urinary infections such as cystitis, urethritis, and prostatitis. Its demulcent properties soothe irritation and inflammation. It is of value for the treatment of enlarged prostate glands and may be used for kidney stones and gravel. As a tonic diuretic, couchgrass has been used with other herbs to treat rheumatism.
Combinations: For urinary tract infections, couchgrass may be used with buchu, bearberry, or yarrow. It can be combined with hydrangea for prostate problems.
Preparations and Dosage: To make a decoction, put 2 teaspoons cut rhizome in 1 cup water, bring to a boil, and simmer 10 minutes. Drink 3 times per day.

As a tincture, take 2–4 ml of the tincture 3 times per day.

CRAMP BARK *(Viburnum opulus* and *Viburnum trilobum)*

Part Used: Bark (dried)
Actions: Anti-inflammatory, antispasmodic, astringent, emmenagogue, hypotensive, nervine
Indications: This herb has a richly deserved reputation as a relaxer of muscular tension and spasm. It has two main uses: for muscular cramps and for ovarian and uterine muscle problems. Cramp bark relaxes the uterus and relieves painful cramps associated with menstrual periods (dysmenorrhea). In a similar way, it may protect against miscarriage.

Its astringent action gives it a role in the treatment of excessive blood loss in menstrual periods and for bleeding associated with menopause.

Preparations and Dosage: To make a decoction, put 2 teaspoons dried herb in a cup of water. Bring to a boil and simmer gently 10–15 minutes. Drink it hot 3 times per day.

As a tincture, take 4–8 ml 3 times per day.

DANDELION *(Taraxacum officinale)*

Parts Used: Root and leaf
Actions: Antirheumatic, bitter, cholagogue, diuretic, hepatic, laxative, tonic
Indications: Dandelion leaf is a very powerful diuretic with effects similar to those of furosemide. But unlike the drug, which can cause a loss of vital potassium from the body, dandelion is a great natural source of potassium. It is an ideally balanced diuretic that may be used safely for cases of water retention due to heart problems. Dandelion root may be used to relieve inflammation and congestion of the liver and gall bladder. It is specific in cases of congestive jaundice. As part of a wider treatment for muscular rheumatism, it can be most effective. This herb is a valuable general tonic and may be the best widely applicable diuretic and liver tonic.

Combinations: For liver and gallbladder problems, dandelion may be used with bearberry or balmony. For water retention, it may be used with couchgrass or yarrow.

Preparations and Dosage: To make a decoction, put 2–3 teaspoons root into 1 cup water, bring to boil, and gently simmer 10–15 minutes. Drink 3 times per day.

As a tincture, take 5–10 ml 3 times per day.

Dandelion leaves may be eaten raw in salads.

DEVIL'S CLAW *(Harpagophytum procumbens)*

Part Used: Rhizome

Actions: Anti-inflammatory, anodyne, hepatic

Indications: This valuable plant is effective for treating some cases of arthritis. This action seems to be due to the presence of a glycoside called harpagoside, which reduces inflammation in the joints. Unfortunately, devil's claw is not always effective, but it is well worth considering whenever arthritis is accompanied by inflammation and pain. This plant also aids in relieving liver and gallbladder symptoms.

Preparations and Dosage: To make a decoction, put ½–1 teaspoon rhizome in 1 cup water. Bring to a boil, then simmer 10–15 minutes. Drink 3 times per day. Use should be continued for at least 1 month.

As a tincture, take 1–2 ml 3 times per day.

ELDER *(Sambucus* spp.)

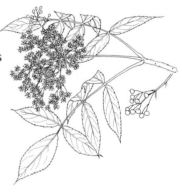

Parts Used: Bark, flowers, berries, leaves

Actions: Bark — diuretic, emetic, purgative; leaves — emollient and vulnerary (externally), diaphoretic, diuretic, expectorant, and purgative (internally); flowers — anticatarrhal, antispasmodic, diaphoretic; berries — diaphoretic, diuretic, laxative

Indications: The elder tree is a medicine chest by itself! The leaves are used for bruises, sprains, wounds, and chilblains. It has been reported that they may be useful in an ointment used for tumors. The flowers are ideal for the treatment of colds and influenza. In fact, they can be used to treat any catarrhal inflammation of the upper respiratory tract, such as that caused by hay fever and sinusitis. Catarrhal deafness responds well to the flowers. Elder berries have properties similar to those of the flowers, and they are useful for treating rheumatism.

Preparations and Dosage: To make an infusion, pour 1 cup boiling water over 2 teaspoons dried or fresh blossoms; steep 10 minutes. Drink hot 3 times per day.

To make a juice, boil fresh berries in water 2–3 minutes, then express the juice. To preserve, add 1 part honey to 10 parts juice; bring to a boil, and then let cool. Take 1 glass diluted with hot water twice per day.

To make an ointment, combine 3 parts fresh elder leaves with 6 parts melted petroleum jelly; heat until the leaves are crisp. Strain and store.

As a tincture, take 2–4 ml 3 times per day.

Caution: The leaves and bark of elder can be poisonous and should be used only as directed. Do not take them internally.

FENUGREEK *(Trigonella foenum-graecum)*

Part Used: Seeds

Actions: Anti-inflammatory, antispasmodic, demulcent, emmenagogue, expectorant, galactogogue, hypotensive, tonic, vulnerary

Indications: For a comprehensive discussion of fenugreek, you must refer to an herbal or materia medica of Ayurvedic medicine. The use of fenugreek in Britain, although limited, demonstrates the value of this herb as a vulnerary; it heals and reduces inflammation in conditions such as wounds, boils, sores, fistulas, and tumors. It can be taken for bronchitis and can be gargled to ease sore throats. Its bitterness explains its role in soothing disturbed digestion. It is a strong stimulator of milk production in mothers, for which it is perfectly safe.

Preparations and Dosage: For external use, the seeds can be pulverized to make a poultice.

To make a decoction to increase milk production, gently simmer 1½ teaspoons seeds in 1 cup water for 10 minutes. Drink 1 cup 3 times per day. Add 1 teaspoon aniseed to make a more pleasant drink.

As a tincture, take 1–2 ml 3 times per day.

FEVERFEW (*Tanacetum parthenium*)

Part Used: Leaves
Actions: Anti-inflammatory, bitter, emmenagogue, vasodilator
Indications: Feverfew has regained its
deserved reputation as a primary remedy
for the treatment of migraine headaches, especially those that are relieved
by applying warmth to the head. It may also help
arthritis during the painful inflammatory stage.
Feverfew can ease dizziness and tinnitus, especially when used
with other remedies, and it relieves painful menstrual periods and
sluggish menstrual flow.

Long-term users of feverfew often report beneficial side
effects, such as relief from depression, nausea, and arthritic pain.
The herb seems to inhibit secretion of the granular contents from
platelets and neutrophils in the blood. This may be relevant to the
therapeutic value of feverfew in migraine and other conditions,
such as osteoarthritis.

AN EXCELLENT HEADACHE REMEDY

Feverfew has been used throughout recorded medical history as a bitter
tonic and remedy for severe headaches. Because of wide media coverage
in recent years, the herb has become known as a "cure" for migraine.
Clinicians at the London Migraine Clinic noted that patients reported
marked improvements when they took the herb. Thankfully, these doc-
tors had the inquiring and open minds of true scientists and started
their own investigations into the claims for feverfew. Pharmacologists
note that it's very likely the sesquiterpene lactones that inhibit pros-
toglandins and histamine, both of which are released during the inflammatory process. In this way, feverfew prevents spasms of the blood
vessels in the head that trigger migraine attacks.

Preparations and Dosage: It's best to eat the equivalent of one fresh leaf 1–3 times per day. Tinctures or tablets are also adequate. When using freeze-dried leaf preparations, take 50–100 mg per day.

Caution: Feverfew should not be used during pregnancy because of its stimulant action on the uterus. The fresh leaves may cause mouth ulcers in sensitive people.

GINGER *(Zingiber officinale)*

Part Used: Rhizome

Actions: Antispasmodic, carminative, diaphoretic, emmenagogue, rubefacient, stimulant

Indications: Ginger may be used as a stimulant of the peripheral circulation in cases of impaired circulation, chilblains, and cramps. In feverish conditions, it acts as a useful diaphoretic, promoting perspiration. As a gargle, it relieves sore throats. Externally, it is the base of many fibrositis and muscle-sprain treatments. Ginger has been used worldwide as an aromatic carminative and pungent appetite stimulant. In India and other countries with hot and humid climates, ginger is eaten daily and is a well-known remedy for digestive problems. Its widespread use is due not only to its flavor but also to its antioxidant and antimicrobial effects.

Preparations and Dosage: To make an infusion, pour 1 cup boiling water over 1 teaspoon fresh root; steep 5 minutes. Drink as needed.

To make a decoction using dried root in powdered or finely chopped form, add 1½ teaspoons to 1 cup water. Bring to a boil, then simmer 5–10 minutes. Drink as needed.

Caution: Do not use ginger during pregnancy or while nursing. Do not consume it if you are also using an antibiotic medication; it may mask toxic symptoms of such therapy. People with gallstones should consult a medical professional before using ginger.

GRAVEL ROOT *(Eupatorium purpureum)*

Parts Used: Rhizome and root

Actions: Antilithic, antirheumatic, diuretic

Indications: Gravel root is used primarily for kidney stones or gravel. It's helpful for urinary infections such as cystitis and urethritis, and it may play a useful role in treating rheumatism and gout.

Preparations and Dosage: To make a decoction, put 1 teaspoon herb in 1 cup water. Bring to a boil, then let simmer 10 minutes. Drink 3 times per day.

As a tincture, take 1–2 ml 3 times per day.

GUAIACUM *(Guaiacum officinale)*

Part Used: Heart-wood

Actions: Anti-inflammatory, antirheumatic, diaphoretic, diuretic, laxative

Indications: Guaiacum is a specific for rheumatic symptoms, including rheumatoid arthritis. It is especially useful for extreme inflammation and pain. It helps treat gout and prevent recurrences of gout. Because of the high content of resins in this valuable herb, it may not be appropriate for people with gastritis or peptic ulceration.

Preparations and Dosage: To make a decoction, put 1 teaspoon wood chips in 1 cup water. Bring to boil, then simmer 15–20 minutes. Drink 3 times per day.

As a tincture, take 1–2 ml 3 times per day.

HOP *(Humulus lupulus)*

Part Used: Flower inflorescence
Actions: Antimicrobial, antispasmodic, astringent, hypnotic, sedative
Indications: Hop has a marked relaxing effect on the central nervous system. It is used extensively to treat insomnia. It eases tension and anxiety and may be used when tension leads to restlessness, headache, or (possibly) indigestion. As an astringent that also has relaxing properties, it can be used for mucous colitis. Hop should, however, be avoided in people with evident depression because it may accentuate this condition. Externally, the antiseptic action of hop is used to treat skin ulcers.
Preparations and Dosage: To make an infusion, pour 1 cup boiling water over 1 teaspoon dried flowers. Infuse 10–15 minutes. Drink 1 cup at night to induce sleep.

As a tincture, take 1–4 ml 3 times per day.

HORSETAIL *(Equisetum arvense)*

Part Used: Aerial stems (dried)
Actions: Astringent, diuretic, vulnerary
Indications: Horsetail is an excellent astringent for the genitourinary system; it reduces hemorrhages and healing wounds because of its high silica content. While it acts as a mild diuretic, its toning and astringent actions make it invaluable for treating incontinence and bedwetting in children. It is considered a specific in cases of inflammation or benign enlargement of the prostate gland. Externally, it is a vulnerary. In some cases, it has been found to ease the pain of rheumatism and stimulate the healing of chilblains.
Preparations and Dosage: To make an infusion, pour 1 cup boiling water over 2 teaspoons dried herb; steep 15–20 minutes. Drink 3 times per day.

To use in a bath to ease rheumatic pain and chilblains: Put 3½ ounces (100 g) herb in hot water; steep 1 hour, then add it to the bath.

As a tincture, take 2–4 ml 3 times per day.

🌿JAMAICAN DOGWOOD *(Piscidia erythrina)*

Part Used: Stem bark

Actions: Anodyne, antispasmodic, nervine

Indications: Jamaican dogwood is a powerful sedative, and in its West Indian homeland it is used as a fish poison. It is not poisonous to humans, but the dosage listed should not be exceeded. It is a powerful remedy for neuralgia and migraine. It can also be used to relieve ovarian and uterine pain. Its main use is for insomnia caused by nervous tension or pain.

Preparations and Dosage: To make a decoction, put 1 teaspoon bark in 1 cup water. Bring to a boil, then simmer gently 10–15 minutes. Drink as needed.

As a tincture, take 1 ml as needed.

🌿KELP *(Fucus vesiculosus)*

Part Used: Whole plant

Actions: Antihypothyroid, antirheumatic

Indications: Kelp has proven very useful for treating underactive thyroid glands and goiter. When obesity is associated with thyroid trouble, kelp may be beneficial because it helps eliminate excess weight. It has a reputation for helping to relieve rheumatism and rheumatoid arthritis when used internally and when applied externally to inflamed joints.

Preparations and Dosage: To make an infusion, pour 1 cup boiling water over 2–3 teaspoons dried herb; steep 10 minutes. Drink 3 times per day.

This herb may also be taken in tablet form as a dietary supplement.

LICORICE *(Glycyrrhiza glabra)*

Part Used: Root (dried)
Actions: Antihepatotoxic, anti-inflammatory, antispasmodic, demulcent, expectorant, mild laxative
Indications: Licorice is a traditional herbal remedy with an ancient history and worldwide use. Modern research has shown that it affects the endocrine system and the liver, among other organs.

Licorice contains triterpenes, constituents that are metabolized in the body to form molecules that have a structure similar to that of the adrenal cortex hormones. This may explain the herb's anti-inflammatory action.

Glycyrrhizin (a triterpene) inhibits the growth of several DNA and RNA viruses, inactivating herpes simplex virus particles irreversibly. It has a wide range of uses in bronchial problems, including catarrh, bronchitis, and coughs in general. Licorice is used in allopathic medicine to treat peptic ulceration. Similarly, herbalists use it to treat gastritis and ulcers. It can be used for relief of abdominal colic.

Preparations and Dosage: To make a decoction, put ½–1 teaspoon root in 1 cup water. Bring to a boil and simmer 10–15 minutes. Drink 3 times per day.

As a tincture take 1–3 ml 3 times per day.

Caution: Avoid prolonged use. Excessive use has been known to promote high blood pressure, cardiovascular toxicity, and edema. Do not use if you have congestive heart failure, kidney disease, diabetes, glaucoma, hypertension, or edema. Do not use during pregnancy, or if you are taking the prescription drug digoxin. There is a small possibility that this herb, when used in large doses, may affect the body's electrolyte balance.

WHAT IS GLYCYRRHIZIN?

Much of the liver-orientated research has focused on the triterpene glycyrrhizin. This substance inhibits hepatocyte injury caused by carbon tetrachloride, benzene hexachloride, and polychlorinated biphenyls (PCBs). As an antihepatotoxic, licorice can be effective in the treatment of chronic hepatitis and cirrhosis, for which it's been widely used in Japan. Glycyrrhizin also enhances antibody production, possibly through the production of interleukin.

LOBELIA *(Lobelia inflata)*

Part used: Aerial parts (dried)
Actions: Antiasthmatic, antispasmodic, emetic, expectorant, nervine
Indications: Lobelia is one of the most useful systemic relaxants available. It has a general depressant action on the central and autonomic nervous system and on neuromuscular action. This herb is used for treating many conditions, often in combination with other herbs. Its primary specific use is for bronchitic asthma and bronchitis.

An analysis of the action of the alkaloids it contains reveals apparently paradoxical effects. Lobeline is a powerful respiratory stimulant, while isolobelanine is an emetic and respiratory relaxant. The herb stimulates catarrhal secretion and expectoration while relaxing the muscles of the respiratory system. The overall action is a truly holistic combination of stimulation and relaxation.
Preparations and Dosage: To make an infusion, pour 1 cup boiling water over ¼ to ½ teaspoons dried leaves; steep 10–15 minutes. Drink 3 times per day.

As a tincture, take ½ ml 3 times per day.
Caution: Do not use during pregnancy. May cause nausea and vomiting. Use dried herb only.

Marsh Mallow *(Althaea officinalis)*

Parts Used: Root and leaf
Actions: Anti-inflammatory, demulcent, diuretic, emollient, expectorant
Indications: Marsh mallow's abundance of mucilage makes this herb an excellent demulcent. The roots have been used mainly to treat the digestive system, while the leaves are used more for the urinary system and lungs.

All inflammatory conditions of the gastrointestinal tract will benefit from the use of marsh mallow. It is helpful for treating inflammations of the mouth, as well as gastritis, peptic ulceration, and colitis. The leaves are beneficial for cystitis, urethritis, urinary gravel, bronchitis, respiratory catarrh, and irritating coughs. Externally, the herb is often used in "drawing" ointments for the treatment of abscesses and boils. It is also applied as an emollient for varicose veins and ulcers.

Preparations and Dosage: Make a cold infusion using the roots by adding 2–4 g root to 1 cup cold water. Steep overnight, then drink.

As a tincture, take 1–4 ml 3 times per day.

Meadowsweet *(Filipendula ulmaria)*

Part Used: Aerial parts
Actions: Antiemetic, anti-inflammatory, antacid, antirheumatic, astringent, carminative
Indications: Meadowsweet is one of the best digestive remedies available. It acts to protect and soothe the mucous membranes of the digestive tract, reducing excess acidity and easing nausea. Used for treating heartburn, hyperacidity, gastritis, and peptic ulcers, meadowsweet's gentle astringency is helpful for diarrhea in children. The presence of aspirin-like chemicals explains

meadowsweet's action in reducing fever and relieving the pain of rheumatism in muscles and joints.

Preparations and Dosage: To make an infusion, pour 1 cup boiling water over 1–2 teaspoons dried herb; steep 10–15 minutes. Drink 3 times per day or as needed.

As a tincture, take 1–4 ml 3 times per day.

MOUNTAIN GRAPE *(Mahonia aquifolia)*

Parts Used: Rhizome and root

Actions: Alterative, anticatarrhal, antiemetic, cholagogue, laxative, tonic

Indications: This herb has actions similar to those of goldenseal and bearberry. It is mainly used for treating chronic and scaly skin conditions, such as psoriasis and eczema. These and other skin conditions are often due to underlying systemic problems; hence, the tonic activity of this herb on the liver and gallbladder may explain its potency. It can be used for stomach and gallbladder conditions, especially those accompanied by nausea and vomiting. As a laxative, it may safely be used for chronic constipation.

Preparations and Dosage: To make a decoction, put 1–2 teaspoons root in 1 cup water. Bring to boil, then simmer 10–15 minutes. Drink 3 times per day.

As a tincture, take 1–4 ml 3 times per day.

MUGWORT *(Artemisia vulgaris)*

Parts Used: Leaves and root

Actions: Bitter tonic, emmenagogue, nervine tonic, stimulant

Indications: Mugwort can be used whenever a digestive stimulant is called for. As a bitter, it stimulates digestive juices and also provides a carminative oil. The herb has a mild nervine action in aiding depression and easing tension. This action is probably due to the volatile oil; thus, care must be taken to protect this oil during preparation. Mugwort may also be used as an emmena-gogue to aid normal menstrual flow.

Preparations and Dosage: To make an infusion, pour 1 cup boiling water over 1–2 teaspoons dried herb; steep 10–15 minutes in a covered container. Drink 3 times per day.

As a tincture, take 1–4 ml 3 times per day.

Mugwort is used as a flavoring in many aperitif drinks — this is a pleasant way to take it!

MUSTARD *(Sinapis alba* and *Brassica nigra)*

Part Used: Seeds

Actions: Diuretic, emetic, irritant, rubefacient, stimulant

Indications: This well-known spice is mainly used as an external stimulant. The rubefacient action causes a mild irritation of the skin, which stimulates circulation in the area and relieves muscular and skeletal pain. Mustard's stimulating diaphoretic action is similar to that of cayenne and ginger.

For relieving fever, colds, and influenza, mustard may be used as a tea or can be ground and sprinkled into a bath. Because it stimulates circulation, it can be helpful for treating chilblains. An infusion or poultice of mustard will ease bronchitis.

Preparations and Dosage: To make a poultice, mix 4 ounces (100 g) freshly ground seeds with warm water to form a thick paste. Spread the paste on a piece of cloth the size of the affected body area. (To prevent the paste from sticking to the skin, lay a damp piece of gauze on the skin.) Apply the poultice and remove after 1 minute. The skin may be slightly irritated by this treatment; apply a bit of olive oil to relieve any irritation.

To make an infusion, pour 1 cup boiling water over 1 teaspoon mustard flour; steep 5 minutes. Drink 3 times per day.

To prepare a foot bath, make an infusion by pouring 2 pints boiling water over 1 tablespoon bruised seeds.

NETTLE *(Urtica dioica)*

Part Used: Aerial parts
Actions: Astringent, diuretic, hypotensive, tonic
Indications: Nettle is an extremely versatile herb. It strengthens and supports the whole body. Throughout Europe it is used as a spring tonic and general detoxifying remedy. In some cases of rheumatism and arthritis, it is astoundingly successful. Nettle is also used as a specific for treating cases of childhood eczema; it's especially useful for nervous eczema. As an astringent, it may be used for nose bleeds or other types of bleeding, including internal bleeding, such as uterine hemorrhage.
Preparations and Dosage: To make an infusion, pour 1 cup boiling water over 1–3 teaspoons dried herb; steep 10–15 minutes. Drink 3 times per day.

As a tincture, take 1–4 ml 3 times per day.
Caution: The fresh herb contains stinging hairs that cause pronounced pain and irritation in the skin. Heat or drying removes this effect.

PARSLEY *(Petroselinum crispum)*

Part Used: Root, leaves, seeds
Actions: Antispasmodic, carminative, diuretic, emmenagogue, expectorant, hypotensive
Indications: The fresh herb, so widely used in cookery, is a rich source of vitamin C. For medicinal purposes, parsley has three main uses. First, it is an effective diuretic, helping rid the body of excess water. Second, it is an emmenagogue, stimulating the menstrual process. (It is advisable not to use parsley in

medicinal dosages during pregnancy because doing so may excessively stimulate the uterus.) Third, as a carminative, it eases flatulence and the colic pains that may accompany it.

Preparations and Dosage: To make an infusion, pour 1 cup boiling water over 1–2 teaspoons leaves or root; steep for 5–10 minutes in a closed container. Drink 3 times per day.

As a tincture, take 1–2 ml 3 times per day.

Caution: Do not use during pregnancy or if you have kidney disease.

POKE *(Phytolacca americana)*

Part Used: Root

Actions: Anticatarrhal, antirheumatic, emetic, purgative, stimulant

Indications: Poke root has a variety of uses and is a valuable addition to many holistic treatments. It's primarily used for treating infections of the upper respiratory tract, removing mucus, and helping cleanse the lymphatic glands. It may be used for tonsillitis, laryngitis, swollen glands, and mumps. This plant is especially valuable for mastitis, for which it's used both internally and as a poultice. Poke root may also be used to treat rheumatism, especially when the condition is long-standing. Used externally as a lotion or ointment, the herb may be used to rid the skin of scabies and other pests.

Preparations and Dosage: To make a decoction, use only small amounts of the herb. Put ¼ teaspoon root in 1 cup water. Bring to a boil, then simmer gently 10–15 minutes. Drink 3 times per day.

As a tincture, take ¼ ml 3 times per day.

Caution: In large doses, poke root is a powerful emetic and purgative.

PRICKLY ASH (*Zanthoxylum americanum*)

Parts Used: Bark and berries

Actions: Alterative, antirheumatic, carminative, circulatory stimulant, diaphoretic, hepatic, tonic

Indications: Prickly ash may be used much as cayenne is, although it is slower in action. It is used in many chronic problems, such as rheumatism and skin diseases. Any sign of poor circulation, such as chilblains, leg cramps, varicose veins, and varicose ulcers, calls for use of this herb. Externally, prickly ash is applied as a stimulating liniment for rheumatism and fibrositis. Because of its stimulating effect on the lymphatic system, circulation, and mucous membranes, it will have a role in the holistic treatment of many different conditions.

Preparations and Dosage: To make an infusion, pour 1 cup boiling water over 1–2 teaspoons dried herb; steep 10–15 minutes. Drink 3 times per day.

As a tincture, take 1–2 ml 3 times per day.

Caution: Do not use during pregnancy.

ROSEMARY (*Rosmarinus officinalis*)

Parts Used: Leaves and twigs

Actions: Antidepressive, antimicrobial, antispasmodic, carminative, emmenagogue rubefacient

Indications: Rosemary is a circulatory and nervine stimulant. It also has a toning and calming effect on digestion when psychological tension is present. It may be used for flatulent dyspepsia, headache, or depression associated with debility.

Externally, it may be applied to ease muscular pain, sciatica, and even neuralgia. It stimulates both the hair follicles and circulation in the scalp, which may be helpful for premature baldness.

Preparations and Dosage: To make an infusion, pour 1 cup boiling water over 1–2 teaspoons dried herb; steep in a covered container 10–15 minutes. Drink 3 times per day.

As a tincture, take 1–2 ml 3 times per day.

SARSAPARILLA *(Smilax officinalis)*

Parts Used: Root and rhizome
Actions: Alterative, antirheumatic, diaphoretic, diuretic
Indications: Sarsaparilla is used for many conditions. As an alterative, it aids proper functioning of the body as a whole. As part of a holistic treatment plan, it helps ease systemic conditions that may lead to rheumatic or skin problems. It is particularly useful for treating psoriasis and other scaly skin conditions, especially when there is irritation. As part of a wider treatment for chronic rheumatism, sarsaparilla should certainly be considered; it's especially useful for rheumatoid arthritis. Finally, research indicates that sarsaparilla contains compounds that aid testosterone activity in the body.

Preparations and Dosage: To make a decoction, put 1–2 teaspoons root in 1 cup water. Bring to a boil, then simmer 10–15 minutes. Drink 3 times per day.

As a tincture, take 1–2 ml 3 times per day.

ST.-JOHN'S-WORT (Hypericum perforatum)

Parts Used: Aerial parts

Actions: Anti-inflammatory, antimicrobial, astringent, nervine, vulnerary

Indications: Taken internally, St.-John's-wort has a sedative and pain-reducing effect. It's helpful for treating neuralgia, anxiety, tension, and similar problems. It is especially useful for menopausal changes that trigger irritability and anxiety. This popular herb is increasingly recommended for treating depression. St.-John's-wort is also helpful for easing fibrositis, sciatica, and rheumatic pain. Externally, it is a valuable healing and anti-inflammatory remedy. As a lotion, it speeds healing of wounds and bruises, varicose veins, and mild burns. The oil is especially useful for the healing of sunburn.

Preparations and Dosage: To make an infusion, pour 1 cup boiling water over 1–2 teaspoons dried herb; steep 10–15 minutes. Drink 3 times per day.

As a tincture, take 2–4 ml 3 times per day.

Caution: Do not use if you are taking antidepressant medication. May cause photosensitization, especially in fair-skinned people.

SWEET VIOLET (Viola odorata)

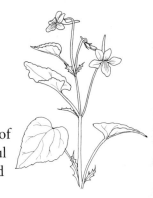

Parts Used: Leaves and flowers

Actions: Expectorant, alterative, anti-inflammatory, diuretic

Indications: Sweet violet has a long history of use as a cough remedy and is especially helpful for the treatment of bronchitis. It may be used to help treat upper respiratory tract catarrh. It is sometimes used for skin conditions such as eczema and to relieve rheumatism. Sweet violet can also be taken to treat urinary infections. This plant has a reputation as an anticancer herb. Whether or not this is true, it definitely has a role in holistic approaches to treating cancer.

Preparations and Dosage: To make an infusion, pour 1 cup boiling water over 1 teaspoon herb; steep 10–15 minutes. Drink 3 times per day.

As a tincture, take 1–2 ml 3 times per day.

WHITE POPLAR *(Populus tremuloides)*

Part Used: Bark
Actions: Anodyne, anti-inflammatory, antiseptic, astringent, bitter tonic, cholagogue
Indications: White poplar is an excellent remedy for arthritis and rheumatism accompanied by severe pain and swelling. For these conditions, its action is quite similar to that of willow; however, it's most effective when used as part of a broad therapeutic approach and not by itself. White poplar can be very helpful for easing flare-ups of rheumatoid arthritis. As a cholagogue, it stimulates digestion and aids stomach and liver function, particularly when there is loss of appetite. It eases feverish colds and treats infections such as cystitis. As an astringent, it may be used for treating diarrhea.

Preparations and Dosage: To make a decoction, put 1–2 teaspoons dried bark in 1 cup water. Bring to a boil, then simmer 10–15 minutes. Drink 3 times per day. To stimulate the appetite, drink the tea 30 minutes before meals.

As a tincture, take 2–4 ml 3 times per day.

WILD CARROT *(Daucus carrota)*

Parts Used: Dried aerial parts and seeds
Actions: Antilithic, antispasmodic, carminative, diuretic
Indications: The volatile oil in wild carrot is an active urinary antiseptic, which helps explain its use for conditions such as cystitis and prostatitis. It has long been considered a specific in the treatment of kidney stones. For treating gout and rheumatism, it is used with other remedies to provide a cleansing diuretic action.

The seeds can be used as a settling carminative agent to relieve flatulence and colic.
Preparations and Dosage: To make an infusion, pour 1 cup boiling water over 1 teaspoon dried herb (or seeds); steep 10–15 minutes. Drink 3 times per day.

As a tincture, take 1–2 ml 3 times per day.
Caution: Do not use wild carrot seeds during pregnancy.

WILD LETTUCE *(Lactuca virosa)*

Part Used: Dried leaves
Actions: Anodyne, antispasmodic, hypnotic, nervine
Indications: At one time, the latex of this herb was sold as "lettuce opium" — an entirely appropriate name, as it turns out. It is a valuable remedy for relieving insomnia, restlessness, and excitability (especially in children) and other manifestations of an overactive nervous system. As an antispasmodic, it can be used as part of a holistic treatment for whooping cough, and for dry, irritated coughs in general. It relieves colic pains in the intestines and uterus, making it useful for dysmenorrhea. It also

eases muscular pains related to rheumatism and has been used as an anaphrodisiac.

Preparations and Dosage: To make an infusion, pour 1 cup boiling water over 1–2 teaspoons herb; steep 10–15 minutes. Drink 3 times per day.

As a tincture, take 1–2 ml 3 times per day.

WILD YAM *(Dioscorea villosa)*

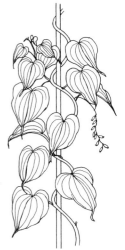

Parts Used: Dried underground parts
Actions: Anti-inflammatory, antirheumatic, antispasmodic, cholagogue, diaphoretic, hepatic
Indications: This valuable herb was at one time the sole source of the chemicals that were used to make contraceptive hormones! In herbal medicine, wild yam relieves intestinal colic, diverticulitis, dysmenorrhea, and ovarian and uterine pains. It is very helpful for treating rheumatoid arthritis, especially in the acute phase, when there is intense inflammation.
Preparations and Dosage: To make a decoction, put 1–2 teaspoons herb in 1 cup water. Bring to a boil, then simmer gently 10–15 minutes. Drink 3 times per day.

As a tincture, take 2–4 ml 3 times per day.

WILLOW *(Salix* spp.)

Part Used: Bark
Actions: Analgesic, anti-inflammatory, tonic
Indications: Willow is an ancient remedy that has been used in various forms for treating rheumatism and gout, fevers, and aches and pains of all kinds. It is usually considered the natural form and origin of modern aspirin.

Preparations and Dosage: To make a decoction, put 1–2 tea-spoons herb in 1 cup water. Bring to a boil, then simmer gently 10–15 minutes. Sip slowly up to 3 times per day.

As a tincture, take 1–4 ml 3 times a day.

YARROW *(Achillea millefolium)*

Parts Used: Aerial parts
Actions: Anti-inflammatory, antimicro-bial, astringent, bitter, diaphoretic, diuretic, hepatic, hypotensive
Indications: Yarrow is one of the best diaphoretic herbs. It's a standard remedy for helping the body cope with fever. It lowers blood pressure through its effects on the peripheral blood vessels, and it stimulates digestion and tones the blood vessels. As a urinary antiseptic, yarrow is helpful for treating conditions such as cystitis. Used externally, yarrow aids in wound healing. It is considered to be a specific for thrombotic conditions associated with high blood pressure.
Preparations and Dosage: To make an infusion, pour 1 cup boil-ing water over 1–2 teaspoons dried herb; steep 10–15 minutes. Drink hot 3 times per day. If you're taking it for fever, drink the infusion every hour.

As a tincture, take 2–4 ml 3 times per day.

YELLOW DOCK *(Rumex crispus)*

Part Used: Root
Actions: Alterative, cholagogue, hepatic, laxative, tonic
Indications: Yellow dock is used extensively for treating chronic skin conditions, such as psoriasis. It contains anthraquinones, which have a significant cathartic action on the bowel. In yellow

dock, however, they seem to act very mildly, possibly because of a tempering effect of the tannin content. Thus, yellow dock is a valuable remedy for constipation because it acts more generally on the body; its actions aren't limited to stimulating the gut muscles. It also promotes the flow of bile and acts as a blood cleanser. Because it acts on the gallbladder, it may be helpful for treating jaundice due to congestion.

Preparations and Dosage: To make a decoction, put 1 teaspoon root in 1 cup water. Bring to a boil, then simmer gently 10–15 minutes. Drink 3 times per day.

As a tincture, take 1–4 ml 3 times per day.

5

MAKING
HERBAL MEDICINES

There is nothing mysterious or even particularly clever about making healing formulations from plants. The pharmaceutical elite would have us think that to be of any use a medicine must be made by a Ph.D. wearing a white lab coat and then packaged with half an acre of rain forest material. Not so! If you can make a cup of tea and cook a meal that your friends would be willing to eat you are qualified. (If this is not the case, or if you've lost friends because of your lack of cooking skills, then perhaps the best place to start is with a book by Julia Child!)

The first way our ancestors used herbs was no doubt by eating the fresh plant. Over the thousands of years that humans have used herbs since then, we have developed other methods of preparing these plants. With our modern knowledge of pharmacology, we can make educated choices about which of these processes to use to release the biochemical constituents that are all-important to healing — without insulting the integrity of the plant by isolating fractions of the whole.

Since healing takes place from within, the most effective way of using herbs is to take them internally. There are numerous ways to prepare internal remedies, but whether you're making a tea, a tincture, or a dry herb preparation, it is essential to work carefully to ensure you end up with what you want.

There are a couple of distinct advantages to making your own herbal medicines. First, you will get a sense of empowerment from being intimately involved in your own healing process. Second, the cost of homemade preparations is many times less than that of commercial medicines.

TEAS

There are two types of herbal teas, or water-based extracts of herbs: infusions and decoctions. There are some basic rules for choosing which method to use with what herb, but, of course, there are many exceptions.

Infusions are the method of choice for non-woody material such as flowers, leaves, and some stems, where the active ingredients are readily accessible. The denser the plant or individual cell walls, the more energy is needed to extract cell contents into the tea; therefore, the more heat-intense process of decocting is used for herbs that contain hard or woody material such as bark, nuts, or roots.

As with anything in the real world, not every herb falls neatly into one of these categories. This is especially true of roots that are rich in volatile oil, such as valerian root. The woodiness of the root suggests decocting, but if the roots are simmered the therapeutically important volatile oil would boil off. Therefore, an infusion is the preparation of choice for valerian root. As you can see, you must learn about the herb you intend to use in order to make the most appropriate preparation.

How to Make an Infusion

If you know how to make tea, you know how to make an infusion. Infusions are best for non-woody parts of the plant such as leaves, flowers, or green stems. If you're making an infusion of bark, root, resin, or seeds, it is best to powder them first to break down some of the cell walls, making them more accessible to water. If you're working with seeds, such as aniseed and fennel, bruise them slightly with a mortar and pestle before infusing to release the volatile oils from the cells. Infuse any aromatic herb, such as chamomile and peppermint, in a well-sealed pot to ensure that only a minimum of the volatile oil is lost through evaporation.

An infusion is the simplest method of utilizing both fresh and dried herbs. Fresh herbs have more water content than dried; when working with fresh herbs, substitute three parts fresh for one part dried. For instance, if the recipe calls for 1 teaspoon of dried herb, substitute 3 teaspoons of fresh herb.

To make an infusion:

Step 1. Warm a china or glass teapot by swishing hot water through it. Place about 1 teaspoon of the dried herb for each cup of tea into the warmed pot.

Step 2. Pour in 1 cup of boiling water for each teaspoon of herb and cover with the lid. Steep for 10 to 15 minutes.

It's usually best to drink medicinal herbal teas hot, but you can drink infusions cold as well. Make a cold infusion if you are working with mucilage-rich herbs, such as marsh mallow, which are sensitive to heat. For a cold infusion, the proportion of herb to water is the same, but let the infusion steep for 6 to 12 hours in a well-sealed pot of cool water. When a hot or cold infusion is ready, strain and sweeten to taste if desired with a bit of honey, brown sugar, or a pinch of a pleasant-tasting herb such as licorice or stevia.

If you prefer not to deal with the messiness of loose leaves, make your own teabags by filling little muslin bags with herbal mixtures (take care to remember how many teaspoons of herb you put into each bag). As with ordinary teabags, pour boiling water over the bag and allow the herbs to steep for 10 to 15 minutes.

Make larger quantities of infusion in the proportion of 1 ounce of herb to 1 pint of water. Whenever possible, infusions should be prepared fresh, but if you do have any leftovers

The Best Herbs for Infusions

Herbal infusions make an exquisite addition to our lifestyles and can open a whole world of subtle delights and pleasures. They are not only medicines or "alternatives" to coffee, but can be delicious beverages in their own right. Everyone will have his or her favorite herbs; here are some of my favorites. Use them individually or in combination. Choose herbs based on both taste and medicinal properties.

Flowers: chamomile, elder flower, hibiscus, linden blossom, red clover

Leaves: lemon balm, lemon verbena, peppermint, rosemary, spearmint

Berries: hawthorn, rose hips

Seeds: aniseed, caraway, celery seed, dill, fennel

Roots: licorice

store them in glass containers in the refrigerator. The shelf life of infusions is not very long; any microorganism that enters the infusion will multiply and thrive in it. If you see any sign of fermentation or spoilage, discard the infusion. These telltale signs can vary, depending on the materials used. Generally, look for color or odor changes, clouding, condensation, and molding; all of these changes indicate spoilage.

How to Make a Decoction

If you select hard, woody herbs, making a decoction will ensure that the soluble contents of the herbs actually reach the water. To ensure that the constituents are transferred to the water, you will need more heat for the decoction process than for infusions.

To make a decoction:

Step 1. In a glass, ceramic, earthenware, or enameled metal pot or saucepan, place 1 teaspoon of dried herb for each cup of water. (For larger quantities, use 1 ounce of dried herb for each pint of water.)

Step 2. Add 1 cup of water for each teaspoon of dried herb. Bring to a boil and then simmer for 10 to 15 minutes or for the amount of time specified for the particular herb or mixture. If the herb contains volatile oils, cover the pot.

Step 3. Strain the herbs from the tea while still hot, sweeten if desired, and drink.

If you're preparing a mixture that contains both soft and woody herbs, prepare separate infusions and decoctions to ensure that the more sensitive herbs are treated accordingly. Combine the two liquids and drink.

TINCTURES

Extracts of herbs in alcohol or glycerin are called tinctures. Tinctures are much stronger, volume for volume, than infusions or decoctions, so the dosage is usually much smaller. Tinctures also have a longer shelf life, extract all of the soluble material from the plant, and tend to be less expensive than other preparations. Tinctures have the benefit of concentration, making them more convenient to take.

Tinctures are used in a variety of ways. You can take one straight or mix it with a cup of cool or hot water. When added to hot water, the alcohol in the tincture will largely evaporate, leaving most of the extract in the water. You can also add a few drops of tincture to a bath or footbath, use it in a compress, mix it with oil and fat to make an ointment, or use it to make suppositories and lozenges.

Wine-Based Tinctures

Another way to make a kind of alcohol tincture is to infuse herbs in wine. Even though these wine-based preparations do not have the shelf life of other tinctures and are not as concentrated, they can be both pleasant to take and effective.

How to Make a Tincture

Alcohol is a better solvent than water for most plant constituents; alcohol dissolves nearly all of the ingredients and acts as a preservative. Tinctures based on glycerin have the advantage of being milder on the digestive tract and are a good bet for people who would rather not ingest alcohol. However, glycerin does not dissolve resinous or oily materials well. As a solvent, glycerin is generally better than water but not as good as alcohol.

The method outlined here is a basic approach. Remember, if you are using fresh rather than dried herbs, use three times the amount. To make a tincture:

Step 1. In a glass container that can be closed tightly, place 4 ounces of finely chopped or ground dried herb. Pour 1 pint of 80-proof vodka over the herbs and cover tightly. If using glycerin as the solvent, make a mixture of ½ pint glycerin and ½ pint water (for fresh herbs, use a mixture of 75 percent glycerin to 25 percent water); pour this mixture over the herbs and cover the container tightly.

Step 2. Keep the container in a warm but dark place for at least 2 weeks and shake it once a day.

Step 3. Strain the liquid through a muslin cloth suspended in a bowl. Wring out all the liquid from the herbs. (The spent herbs make excellent compost!)

Step 4. Pour the tincture into a dark glass bottle. Close the bottle tightly and label with all ingredients and the date. Stored properly out of direct sunlight, the tincture will last many years.

DRY HERB PREPARATIONS

There a number of advantages to taking herbs in a dry form, mainly because you can avoid the taste of the herb while consuming the whole herb (including the woody material). Unfortunately, there are also a number of drawbacks:

- Dry herbs are unprocessed, and so the constituents are not always readily available for easy absorption. Unlike an infusion, during which heat and water help to break down the walls of the plant cells and dissolve the constituents, the digestive process of the stomach and small intestines is not guaranteed to break down plant cell walls.
- When the herb's constituents are already dissolved in liquid form, they are available a lot more quickly and begin their action sooner.
- Avoiding the taste of the herb can also be considered a drawback. For instance, bitter herbs work best when tasted, since their effects result from a neurological reflex. When bitters are put into a capsule or a pill, their action can be diminished or even lost.

Taking all these considerations into account, there are a number of ways to use herbs in dry form. Always be sure the herbs are powdered as finely as possible. Grinding guarantees that the cell walls are largely broken down and helps in the digestion and absorption of the herb.

The most convenient way to grind herbs is with a coffee or spice grinder; don't use the same one for your coffee or spices, as it can retain the scent and flavor of the herbs. Mortars and pestles are traditional options and look more attractive, but they sometimes require hard work to use. For larger quantities of herbs, a food processor is ideal.

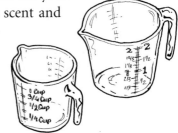

Capsules

Gelatin capsules are a convenient way to use powdered herbs. The capsule size depends on the amount of herbs prescribed per dose, the density of the plant, and the volume of the material. A size 00 capsule, for instance, holds about ⅙ ounce of finely powdered herb.

Filling a capsule is easy:

Step 1. Place the powdered herbs on a flat dish and separate the halves of the capsule.

Step 2. Move the halves of the capsules through the powder, scooping the herb into the two halves.

Step 3. Push the halves of the capsule together.

Capsules should be stored in a sealed container in a cool, dry place out of direct sunlight. This type of medicine is usually best taken with food, but the specifics will vary from herb to herb.

Pills

There are a number of ways to make pills, from the very simple to the complex. The simplest way to take an unpleasant remedy is to place the powder on a slice of fresh bread. Roll into a small ball shape. This method works most effectively with herbs such as goldenseal or cayenne.

GLOSSARY

Analgesic. A medication or treatment that relieves pain.

Ankylosing spondylitis. A rheumatic disease that causes arthritis of the spine and sacroiliac joints. Occasionally may cause inflammation of the eyes and heart valves.

Antibodies. Special proteins produced by the body's immune system that recognize and help fight infectious agents, such as bacteria or other foreign substances that invade the body. Should abnormal antibodies develop, they may attack a part of the body, causing an autoimmune disease. These abnormal antibodies are called autoantibodies.

Antigen. A foreign substance that stimulates an immune response.

Antinuclear antibodies. Abnormal antibodies that are often present in people with connective tissue diseases or other autoimmune disorders.

Arthritis. Literally means joint inflammation. It is a general term for more than 100 conditions known as rheumatic diseases. Some of these diseases affect not only the joints, but also other parts of the body, including important supporting structures such as muscles, tendons, and ligaments, as well as some internal organs.

Bacteria. Any group of single-celled microorganisms. Bacteria live in soil, water, and organic matter and in the bodies of plants, animals, and humans. Some types of bacteria cause illness when they enter the body; others are benign or even beneficial.

Bursa (plural, bursae). A small sac of tissue located between bones and other moving structures, such as muscles, skin, or tendons. The bursae contain a lubricating fluid that allows adjoining structures to glide smoothly back and forth.

Bursitis. A condition involving inflammation of the bursae.

Cartilage. A tough, resilient tissue that covers and cushions the ends of the bones and absorbs shock.

Colchicine. A medicine used to treat gout. It may be given by mouth (orally) or injected directly into a vein (intravenously).

Collagen. The main structural protein of skin, bones, tendons, cartilage, and connective tissue.

Connective tissue. The supporting framework of the body and its internal organs.

Corticosteroids. Potent anti-inflammatory hormones that are made naturally in the body, or which are created synthetically for use as drugs. The most commonly prescribed drug of this type is prednisone.

Crystal-induced arthritis. An accumulation of crystalline material in various parts of the body, especially the joints. Gout and pseudogout are examples of crystal-induced arthritis.

Enteric. A general term that refers to the intestines and the digestion of food.

Erythrocyte sedimentation rate. A blood test that measures the speed at which red blood cells settle at the bottom of a test tube. A high rate signals possible inflammatory disease. Also referred to as the "sed" rate, or the "ESR."

Fibromyalgia. A chronic disorder characterized by widespread musculoskeletal pain, fatigue, and tenderness in localized areas of the neck, spine, shoulders, and hips. These painful areas are called tender points.

Fibrous capsule. A tough wrapping of tendons and ligaments that surrounds the joints.

Gastrointestinal tract. Organs related to the digestion of food, including the stomach and the intestines.

Glycosaminoglycan (GAG). Very large molecules made up of amino sugars. These are spongy, water-holding molecules that form the gel-like matrix of ground substance. They are found in all connective tissue and mucous membranes. Glucosamine macromolecules are the basic substrate of cartilage, ligaments, tendons, and bones

Gout. A type of arthritis resulting from deposits of needlelike crystals of uric acid in the connective tissue, joint spaces, or both. The body's reaction to the crystals causes inflammation and extreme pain in the affected joint, most commonly the big toe. Gout is caused by either increased production of uric acid or failure of the body to eliminate uric acid.

HLA-B27. A genetic marker that may be found in the blood of patients with certain forms of arthritis, such as ankylosing spondylitis and Reiter's syndrome.

Hydrotherapy. Therapy that takes place in water.

Hyperuricemia. Increased amount of uric acid in the blood.

Immunosuppressive drugs. Medicines that decrease the immune response and may relieve some symptoms of severe Reiter's syndrome and a variety of autoimmune disorders.

Infectious arthritis. Forms of arthritis caused by infectious agents, such as bacteria or viruses.

Inflammation. A characteristic reaction of tissues to injury or disease. It is marked by four signs: swelling, redness, heat, and pain.

Joint. The place where two or more bones are joined. Most joints are composed of cartilage, joint space, fibrous capsule, synovium, and ligaments.

Joint space. The area enclosed within the fibrous capsule and synovium.

Juvenile arthritis. A term used to refer to the types of arthritis that affect children. Juvenile rheumatoid arthritis is the most common type.

Ligaments. Bands of cordlike tissue that connect bone to bone.

Lupus. A type of immune disorder known as an autoimmune disease. It can lead to inflammation of and damage to joints, skin, kidneys, heart, lungs, blood vessels, and brain.

Lyme disease. A disease caused by the bacterium *Borrelia burgdorferi*. Arthritis is often a prominent symptom. Rash, heart disease, and nervous system involvement may also occur.

Manipulation. A treatment in which health professionals use their hands to help restore normal movement to stiff joints.

Mobilization therapies. A group of treatments that include traction, massage, and manipulation. When performed by a trained professional, these methods can help control pain and increase joint and muscle motion.

Nonsteroidal anti-inflammatory drug (NSAID). A group of drugs that includes aspirin and aspirin-like drugs such as ibuprofen and acetaminophen. NSAIDs are used to reduce the inflammation that causes joint pain, stiffness, and swelling. As the name suggests, NSAIDs do not contain corticosteroids.

Osteoarthritis. A type of arthritis that causes cartilage in the joints to fray and wear. In extreme cases, the cartilage may wear away completely.

Polymyositis. A rheumatic disease that causes weakness and inflammation of muscles.

Pseudogout. Similar to gout. However, the crystals in the synovial fluid are composed of calcium pyrophosphate dihydrate and not uric acid. As with gout, the crystals in the joint space cause an intense inflammatory reaction.

Psoriatic arthritis. Joint inflammation that occurs in about 5 to 10 percent of people with psoriasis (a common skin disorder).

Purines. Components of all human tissue that break down to form uric acid. Purines are also found in many foods.

Range of motion. A measurement of the extent to which a joint can go through all of its normal movements.

Reactive arthritis. A form of arthritis that develops after an infection involving the lower urinary tract, bowel, or other organs.

Rheumatic. A term referring to a disorder or condition that causes pain or stiffness in the joints, muscles, or bones.

Rheumatic diseases. A general term that refers to more than 100 conditions that affect joints, muscles, bones, and other connective tissues.

Rheumatoid arthritis. A chronic inflammatory disease that causes pain, stiffness, swelling, and loss of function in the joints. The primary target of rheumatoid arthritis is the synovium, or joint lining. This tissue, which normally is smooth and shiny, becomes inflamed, painful, and swollen. The disease can also cause inflammation in the blood vessels and the outer lining of the heart and lungs.

Rheumatoid factor. A special kind of antibody often found in people with some types of rheumatic diseases.

Rheumatologist. A doctor who specializes in diagnosing and treating disorders that affect the joints, muscles, tendons, ligaments, and bones.

Risk factor. Something that increases a person's chance of developing a disease, such as age, gender, ethnicity, and genetics (family history).

Sacroiliitis. Inflammation of the sacrum.

Sacrum. The part of the spine that connects to the pelvis.

Scleroderma. A disease of the connective tissues and blood vessels that leads to hardening of the skin. Scleroderma can also damage internal organs such as the kidneys, lungs, heart, or gastrointestinal tract.

Spondylitis. Inflammation of the vertebrae.

Synovial fluid. Fluid released into movable joints by surrounding membranes. The fluid lubricates the joints and reduces friction during movement.

Synovium. A thin membrane that lines a joint and releases a fluid that allows the joint to move easily.

Tendinitis. Inflammation of tendons caused by overuse, injury, or other rheumatic conditions.

Tendons. Fibrous cords of tissue that connect muscle to bone.

Tophus (plural, tophi). A hard deposit of crystalline uric acid that may appear as a lump just under the skin, particularly around the joints and at the rim of the ear.

Transcutaneous. Through the skin.

Urethritis. Inflammation of the urethra, the canal that carries urine away from the bladder. (In males, the urethra also carries semen.)

Uric acid. An organic substance that results from the breakdown of purines or waste products in the body. Most people with gout have high levels of uric acid in the blood. If the concentration of uric acid in the tissues rises above normal levels, crystals can form in the joints and cause inflammation.

Urogenital tract. Organs related to the production and excretion of urine, and to reproduction.

RESOURCES

American Chronic Pain Association
800-533-3231
www.theacpa.org
The association provides information on positive ways
to deal with chronic pain and can provide guidelines
on selecting a pain management center.

American College of Rheumatology/
Association of Rheumatology Health Professionals
404-633-3777
www.rheumatology.org
The association provides referrals to rheumatologists
and physical and occupational therapists who have
experience working with people with rheumatic diseases. The organization also provides educational
materials and guidelines about many different
rheumatic diseases.

Arthritis Foundation
800-283-7800
www.arthritis.org
The main voluntary organization devoted to arthritis. The foundation publishes free pamphlets on many types of arthritis, and also a monthly magazine for members, which provides up-to-date information. The foundation can also provide physician and even clinic referrals. Their store also carries videos targeting individuals with arthritis.

Fibromyalgia Network
800-853-2929
http://fmnetnews.com
An organization that provides information about this painful condition. It publishes newsletters and provides informational pamphlets.

National Institute of Arthritis and Musculoskeletal and Skin Diseases
National Institutes of Health, Department of Health and Human Services
877-226-4267
www.niams.nih.gov
This clearinghouse provides information about various forms of arthritis and rheumatic diseases. The clearinghouse distributes patient and professional educational materials and also refers people to other sources of information.

National Institute on Aging
National Institutes of Health, Department of Health and Human Services
800-222-4225
www.nia.nih.gov
Strives to understand the nature of aging in order to extend the healthy, active years of life.

National Osteoporosis Foundation
800-231-4222
www.nof.org
One of the nation's leading voluntary health organizations dedicated to osteoporosis and bone health. Provides programs of awareness, education and training, advocacy and research.

Spondylitis Association of America
800-777-8189
www.spondylitis.org
A non-profit voluntary organization helping people who have ankylosing spondylitis and related conditions. It sells books and DVDs about exercises for people with arthritis of the spine.

INDEX

Page numbers in *italics* indicate illustrations.

OTHER STOREY TITLES YOU WILL ENJOY

Hands-On Healing Remedies, by Stephanie Tourles.
150 herbal recipes for balms, salves, oils, liniments and other topical
therapies for everyday skin conditions and body ailments.
320 pages. Paper. ISBN 978-1-61212-006-5.

Herbal Antibiotics, 2nd edition, by Stephen Harrod Buhner.
The essential guide to building your natural defenses using
herbal alternatives to standard antibiotics.
480 pages. Paper. ISBN 978-1-60342-987-0.

The Herbal Home Remedy Book, by Joyce A. Wardwell.
A wealth of herbal healing wisdom, with advice on how to collect
and store herbs, make remedies, and stock a home herbal medicine chest.
176 pages. Paper. ISBN 978-1-58017-016-1.

Rosemary Gladstar's Herbal Recipes for Vibrant Health.
A practical compendium of herbal lore and know-how for wellness,
longevity, and boundless energy.
408 pages. Paper. ISBN 978-1-60342-078-5.

Rosemary Gladstar's Herbal Remedies for Children's Health.
How to use herbs such as chamomile, lemon balm, and echinacea to create
gentle baby care products and safe treatments for childhood illnesses.
80 pages. Paper. ISBN 978-1-58017-153-3.

Rosemary Gladstar's Medicinal Herbs: A Beginner's Guide.
How to grow, harvest, prepare, and use 33 of the most common
and versatile healing plants.
224 pages. Paper. ISBN 978-1-61212-005-8.

These and other books from Storey Publishing are available
wherever quality books are sold or by calling 1-800-441-5700.
Visit us at *www.storey.com* or sign up for our newsletter
at *www.storey.com/signup.*